TYPE 2 DIABETES

Cookbook

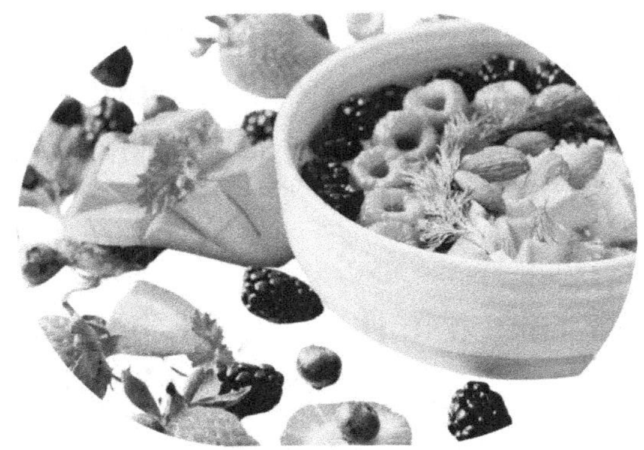

Budget-friendly, Quick & Easy Recipes for Newly Diagnosed Type 2 Warriors with a 4-Week Meal Plan

Allison D. Dixon

Copyright

©

2024 Allison D. Dixon

Disclaimer:

The information presented in this cookbook is for educational and informational purposes only. While every effort has been made to ensure the accuracy and completeness of the content, the author and publisher assume no responsibility for errors or omissions or for any damages resulting from the use of the information contained herein.

Readers are strongly advised to consult with a qualified health practitioner before making any dietary or lifestyle changes based on the content of this cookbook. The author and publisher disclaim any liability arising directly or indirectly from the use of this cookbook.

Any trademarks, service marks, product names, or named features are assumed to be the property of their respective owners and are used only for reference. There is no implied endorsement if such names are mentioned.

Thank you for respecting the intellectual property and legal rights associated with this cookbook.

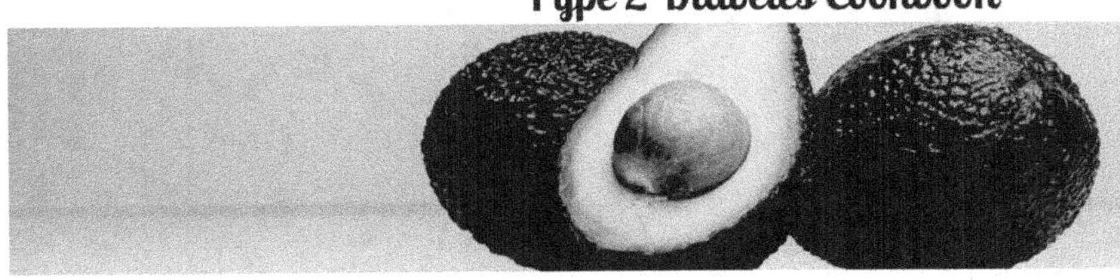

PREFACE

Hello, my name is Allison D. Dixon, and I am excited to share this adventure with you. Before we get started on delicious and diabetes-friendly dishes, allow me to pull back the curtain a little. You see, this cookbook, like the others I've published and those in the works, is the result of my personal experiences as a dietician and a daughter.

My mother's journey with type 2 diabetes changed the course of my life. It was one of those life-changing experiences that left an indelible impression. The same recipes you're about to discover accompanied her

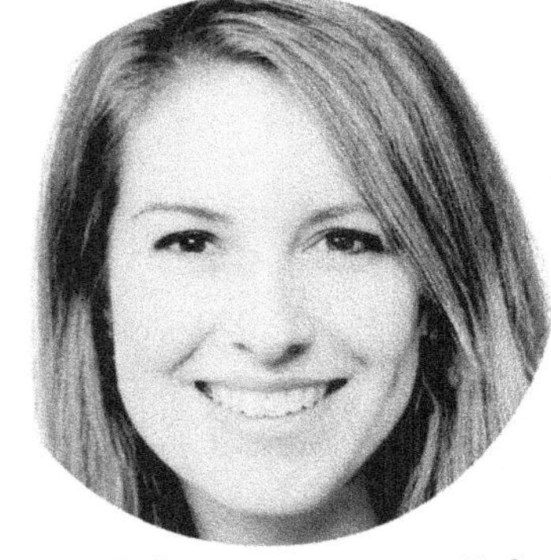

on this voyage. It's more than just a list of ingredients and directions; it's a story of triumph over adversity, one that countless others have adopted.

Consider this: family gatherings filled with laughter, the aroma of nutritious meals wafting through the kitchen, and a sense of empowerment as my mother not only controlled her disease but enjoyed life to the fullest. These recipes have been a lifeline for many people, not just those with type 2 diabetes, but also those suffering from type 1.

So, as we go on this culinary trip together, remember that these dishes are more than simply food; they're about rediscovering joy, relishing life, and finding strength in each meal.

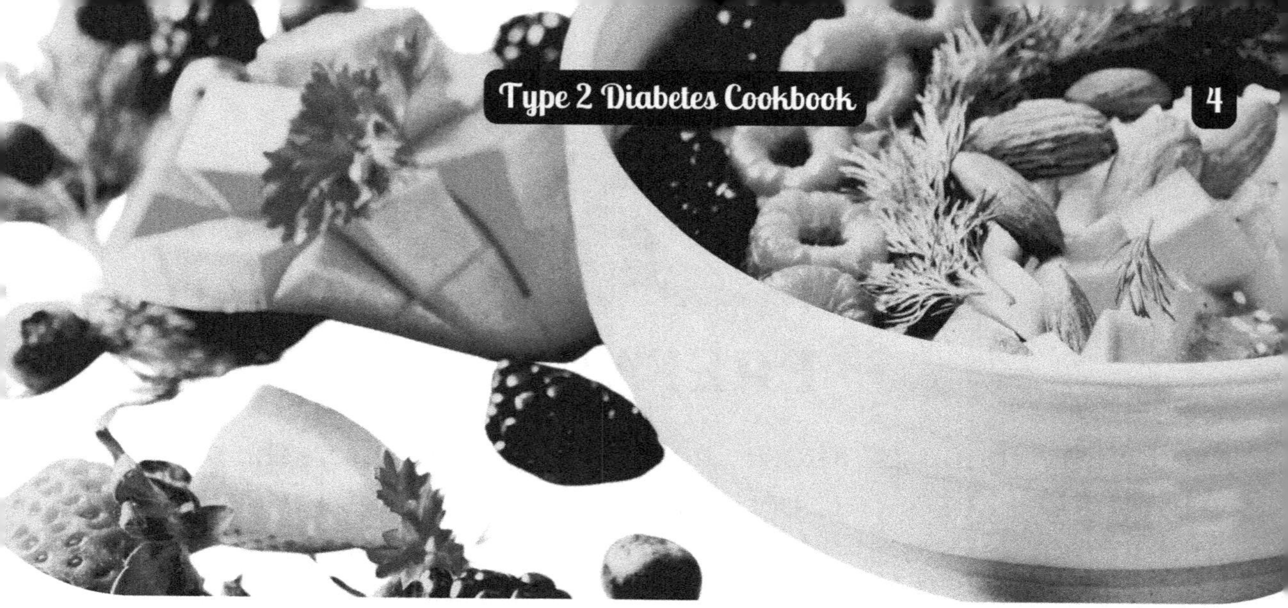

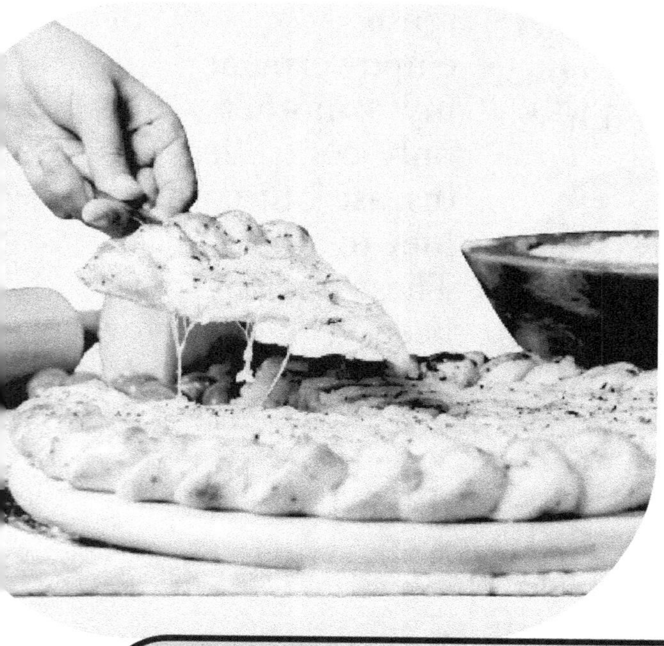

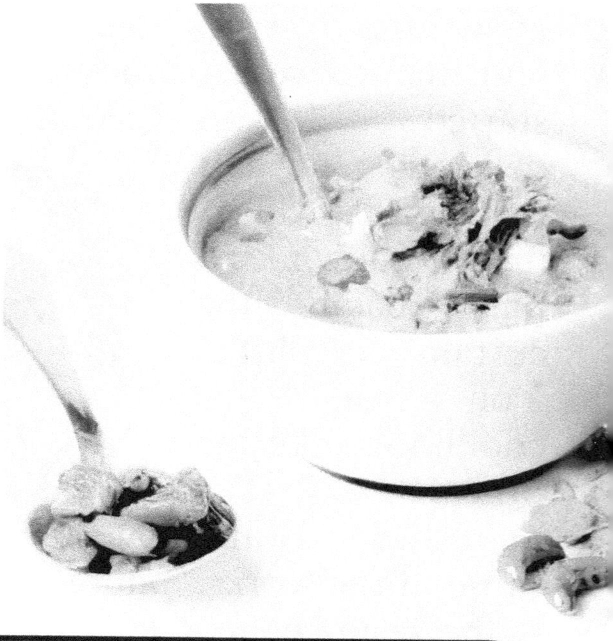

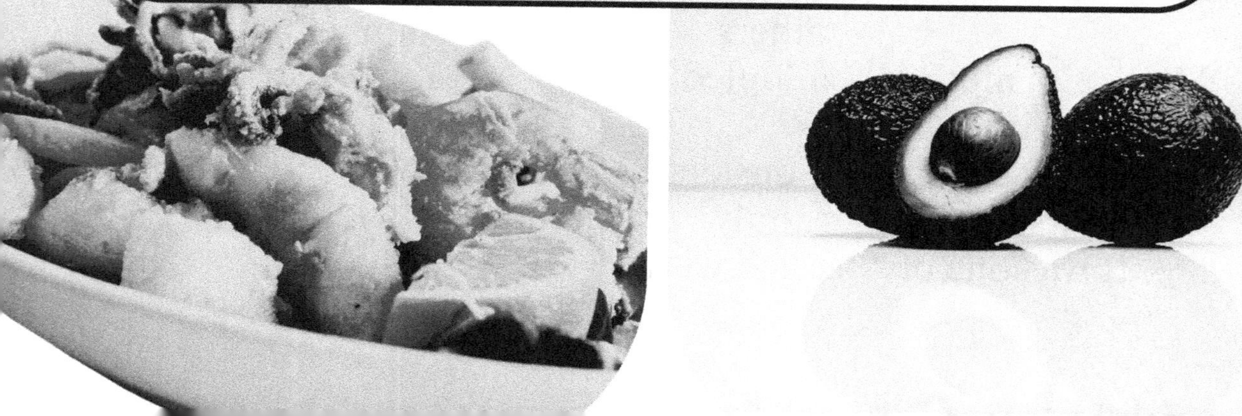

Nourishing Choices: A Symphony of Diabetes-Friendly Delights. Balancing flavor, health, and joy on every plate. #DiabetesFriendlyEats

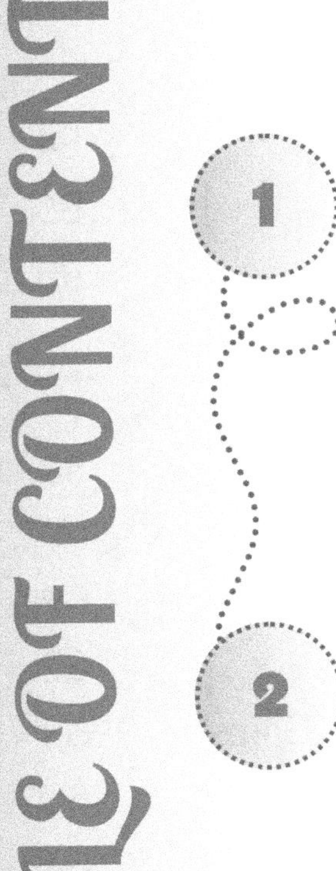
TABLE OF CONTENTS

TABLE OF CONTENTS

INTRODUCTION

Understanding Type 2 Diabetes

Let's clear up the confusion surrounding Type 2 Diabetes. It works like this: our bodies normally convert the food we eat into glucose, a sugar that serves as fuel for our cells. Insulin, a pancreatic hormone, facilitates the transport of glucose into our cells for energy production.

Things get a little out of control when you have Type 2 Diabetes. Either the pancreas does not produce enough insulin, or the body does not use it efficiently - it's as if the key (insulin) can't quite unlock the door (cells) to allow glucose in.

Imagine insulin as a superhero attempting to allow glucose to enter the cells. In Type 2 Diabetes, either the superhero is slacking off or the door does not open properly. What was the result? Glucose accumulates in the blood, creating a rise in blood sugar levels.

So, what causes this? Lifestyle factors, such as food, exercise, and heredity, all play an important impact. Being a couch potato and bingeing on processed foods? That may nudge you towards Type 2 Diabetes.

Now, about the symptoms: they can be subtle. Frequent thirst, unexpected weight loss, and fatigue are all warning flags indicating that something isn't quite right. But here's the catch: Type 2 Diabetes can occasionally go undetected, brewing in the background.

The good news is that Type 2 Diabetes can be managed. You may be the captain of your own health ship by making the necessary lifestyle adjustments, engaging in physical activity, and eating a well-balanced and nutritious diet.
Now I understand - it may seem like a lot, but knowledge is power.

Understanding what is happening in your body is the first step toward gaining control. So, while we work through this cookbook together, consider it your guide to making those powerful decisions, one delicious food at a time.
Stay tuned for more advice and delicious snacks.

Importance of Diet in Diabetes Management

Let's talk about why your diet is a game changer for treating diabetes, particularly Type 2. Consider your body to be a well tuned machine, with food serving as the fuel to keep it working properly. Now that diabetes has entered the picture, it's as if we're designing that fuel to be both super-efficient and diabetes-friendly.

The simple truth is that what you eat has a direct impact on your blood sugar levels. Different meals affect your body in unique ways. Carbohydrates, for example, are converted into sugar, leading your blood sugar to rise. Proteins and fats also play a role, albeit with a slower and softer effect.

Now, I am not here to preach deprivation. No, that's not the feeling. It's all about finding the right balance and making choices that help your body work with insulin. Imagine this: You have a plate, and you are the artist. Fill it with a variety of vegetables, lean proteins, whole grains, and some healthy fats. It's not just about controlling your blood sugar; it's also about nourishing your body, strengthening it, and providing it with the resources it needs to beat diabetes.

And let's talk about portions; it's like Goldilocks and the Three Bears. Not too much, not too little—just right. This helps prevent blood sugar swings. Don't forget the hydration dance. Water is your buddy, helping you flush off extra sugar and keep things running smoothly.

Now I understand. Life is hectic, and sometimes the drive-thru or a bag of chips feels like the only alternative. But don't worry, we're going to make healthy eating easy, pleasant, and a natural part of your lifestyle.

This cookbook is not about strict guidelines. It's about delicious, gratifying meals that are also very good for your blood sugar. So, let's dig into these dishes and transform your kitchen into a health oasis.

Cheers to a platter full of deliciousness!

Tips for Navigating a Diabetic-Friendly Kitchen

Hey Kitchen Maverick,
Creating a diabetic-friendly kitchen is like setting up your culinary haven for success. Let's break it down into some nifty tips to make your kitchen the ultimate ally in your diabetes journey.

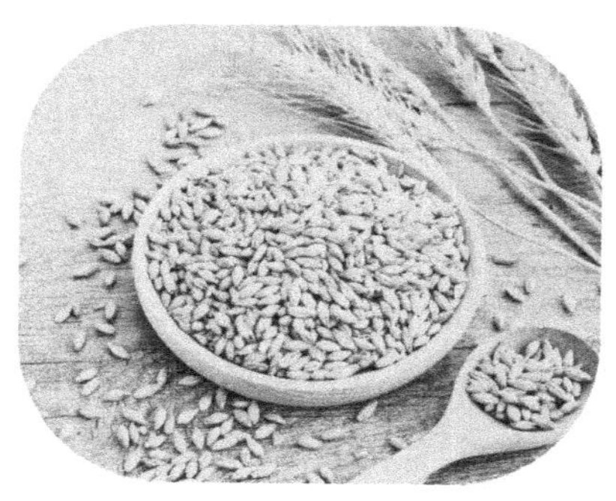

1. Stock Up on Smart Carbs:
Swap refined grains for whole grains like brown rice, quinoa, and whole wheat. These complex carbs are the heroes that keep your blood sugar in check.

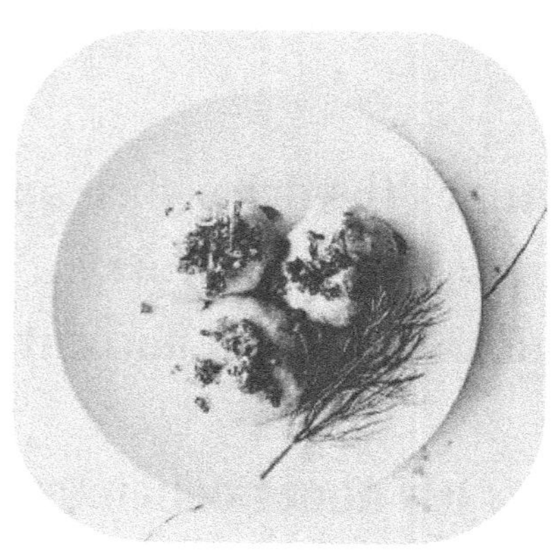

2. Master the Art of Portion Control:
Invest in measuring cups and spoons. They're like your kitchen wingmen, ensuring you're not overloading your plate with more than you bargained for.

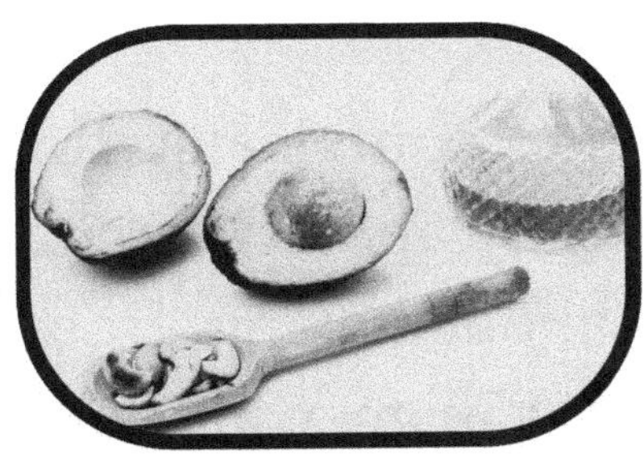

3. **Embrace Healthy Fats**:

Olive oil, avocados, and nuts – these are your kitchen VIPs. They bring the good fats to the table, promoting heart health and satiety.

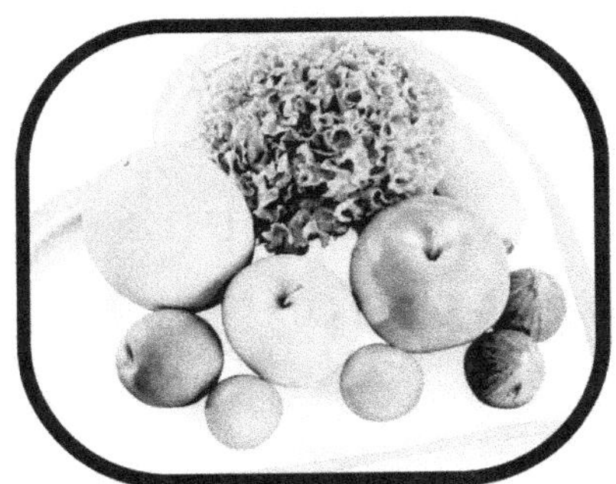

4. **Build a Veggie Wonderland**:

Make veggies the stars of your meals. Fresh, frozen, or canned (just watch the sodium), veggies add a burst of flavor, nutrition, and color to your plate.

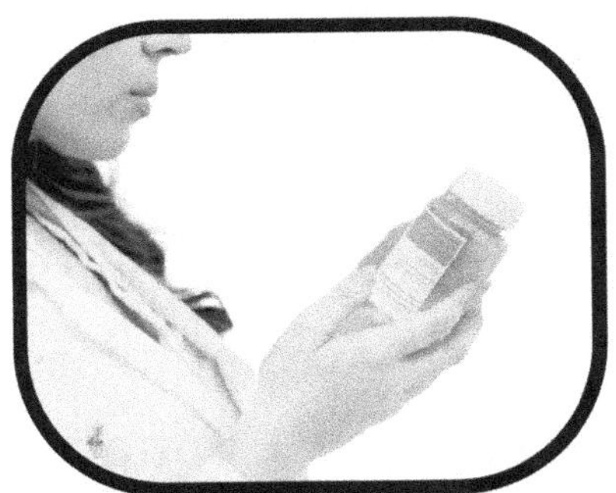

5. **Label Love**:

Get friendly with food labels. Look out for hidden sugars and sneaky carbs. The more you know, the more empowered your choices become.

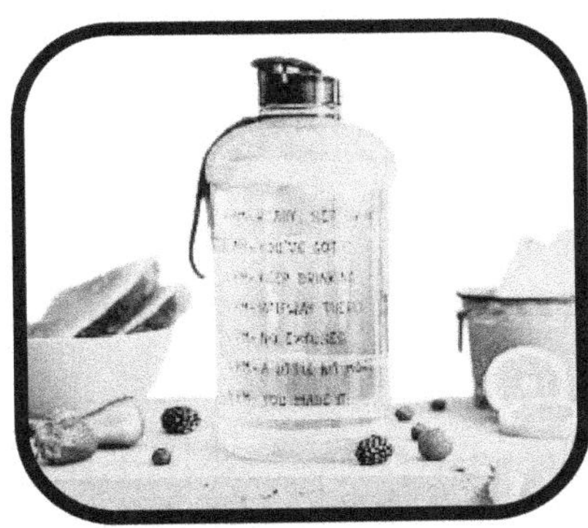

6. **Hydration Station**:

Water is your kitchen's unsung hero. Keep a water bottle handy, reminding you to stay hydrated and helping flush out excess sugar.

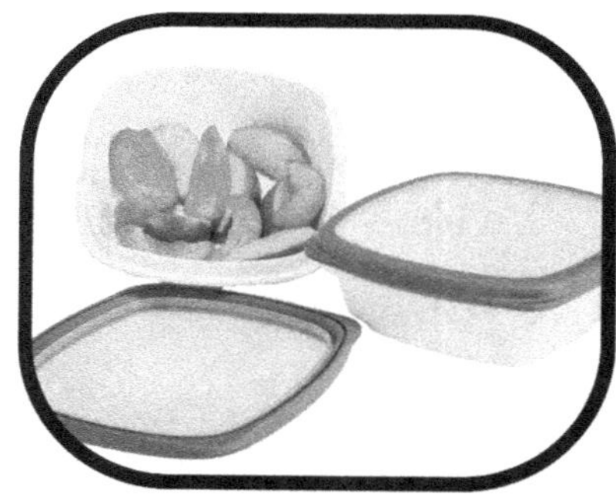

7. **Mindful Storage**:
Invest in airtight containers for leftovers. It's not just about keeping things fresh; it's about having grab-and-go options that align with your diabetes-friendly goals.

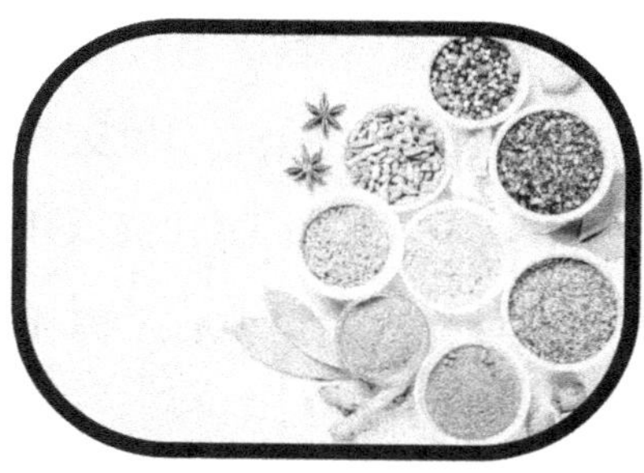

8. **Herb and Spice Symphony**:
Ditch the salt shaker and turn to herbs and spices for flavor. They're like the maestros of taste without the blood pressure spike.

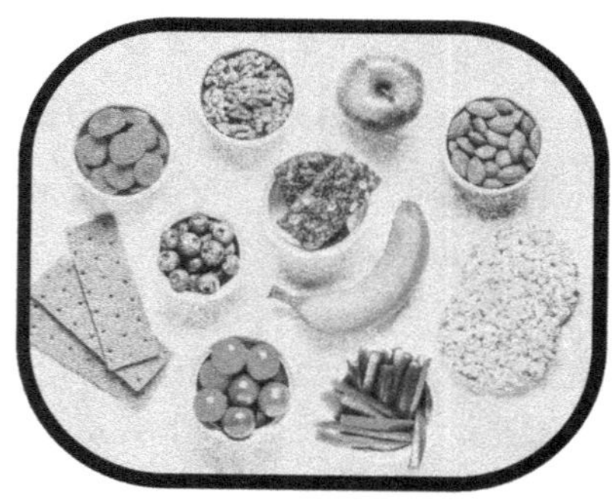

9. **Smart Snacking Solutions**:
Create a snack haven with options like nuts, seeds, and veggies with hummus. Bid farewell to mindless munching and welcome mindful snacking.

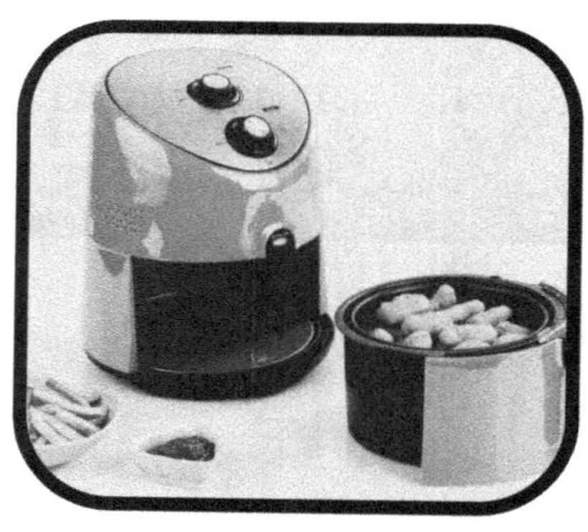

10. **Gadget Galore**:
Consider investing in kitchen gadgets that make life easier – think spiralizers for veggie noodles or an air fryer for crispy, guilt-free delights.

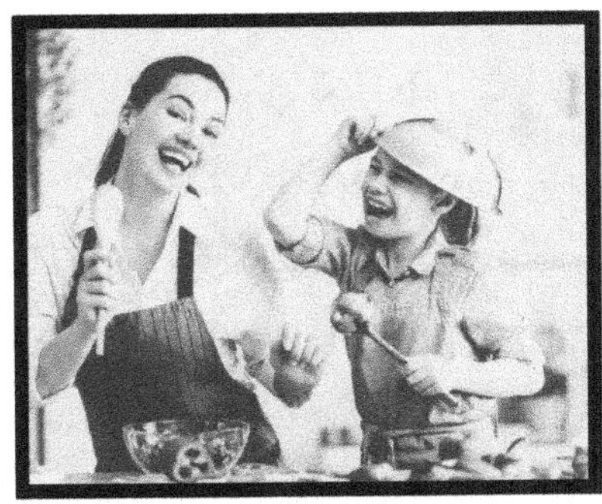

11. Educate Your Kitchen Crew:
Share the love with your family or roommates. Educate them on the diabetes-friendly ways of your kitchen, making it a supportive environment for everyone.

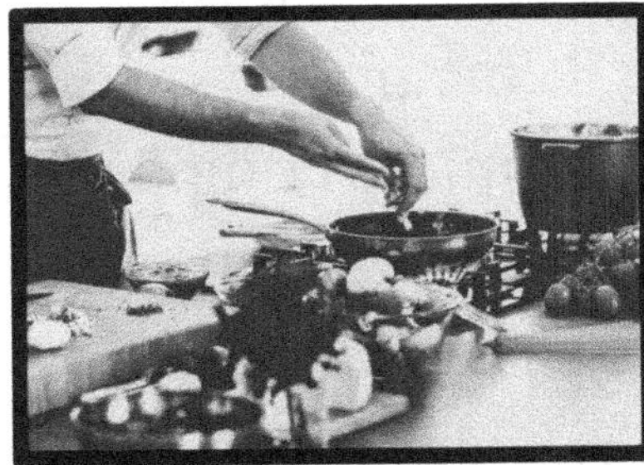

12. Cook with Curiosity:
Be open to trying new recipes and ingredients. Your kitchen is a playground, and experimenting with flavors keeps things exciting.

Your kitchen is your ally, your partner in this journey. By setting it up with these tips, you're not just cooking; you're crafting a lifestyle that supports your health and happiness. Here's to your kitchen becoming the heart of your diabetes-friendly adventure!

Encouragement of a Sustainable and Enjoyable Diabetic Lifestyle:

Embarking on a diabetic path may appear scary at first, but I am confident that with the correct tools, information, and support, it can be a fulfilling and enjoyable trip. As a dietician who has seen the transformative effect of mindful eating, I encourage you to adopt the following principles:

1. **Celebrate Small Victories**: Every positive move you make toward a better lifestyle is a success. Celebrate minor victories, such as trying a new recipe, incorporating more vegetables into your meals, or discovering a fun physical activity.

2. **Listen to Your Body**: Your body is an excellent advisor. Pay attention to how certain foods impact you, and allow that knowledge influence your decisions. Remember that this cookbook is only a tool; your body is the ultimate compass.

3. **Create a Support System**: Whether it's friends, family, or an online community, having a support system may make a huge impact. Share your experience, get advice, and support others on a similar path.

4. **Embrace diversity**: One of the benefits of cooking is the limitless diversity it provides. Experiment with various ingredients, cuisines, and culinary methods. Variety not only keeps meals interesting, but it also provides a varied spectrum of nutrients.

5. **Prioritize Self-Care:** Managing diabetes involves more than simply what you eat; it's also about how you take care of yourself. Prioritize self-care, whether through relaxation techniques, regular exercise, or just dedicating time to activities you enjoy.

6. **Engage Your Senses**: Before taking the first bite, take a moment to appreciate the visual appeal, aroma, and textures of your meal. Engaging your senses enhances the overall eating experience and fosters a deeper connection with your food.

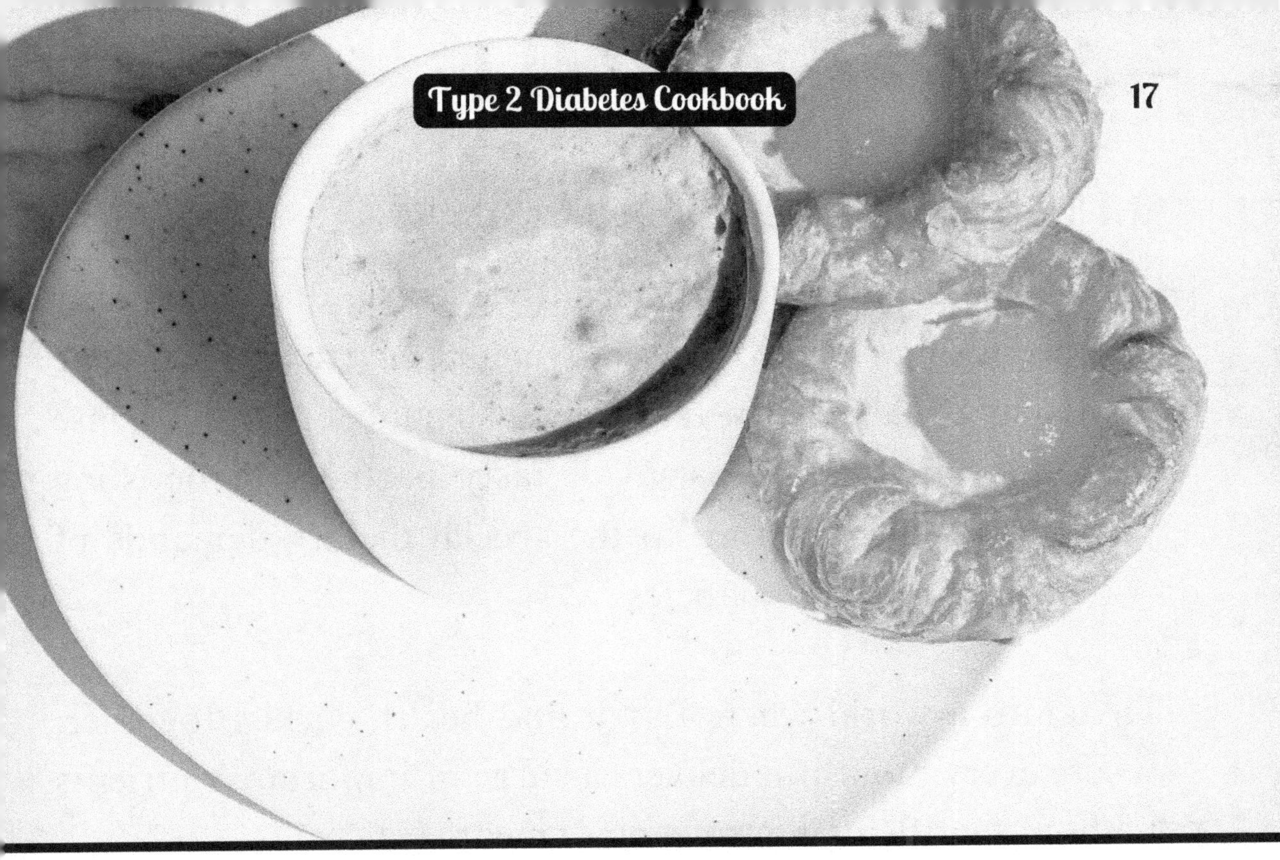

CHAPTER 1
DIABETIC BREAKFASTS

Breakfast, the first meal of the day, deserves to be a culinary symphony as well as a nutritional powerhouse. In this chapter, we'll go over how to make delicious diabetic-friendly breakfasts that will not only get you started in the morning but also help you manage your Type 2 diabetes. From vivid smoothie bowls to cozy overnight oats, these dishes are intended to make your mornings not just healthful but also enjoyable.

1.1 Nutrient-Packed Smoothie Bowls

Embarking on a road to a healthy lifestyle does not imply compromising taste or enjoyment, particularly while controlling diabetes. In terms of sustenance, nutrient-dense smoothie bowls serve as vivid, tasty partners in boosting well-being while catering to the special dietary demands of persons dealing with diabetes.

Dive into a world where flavor and health coexist together, where every mouthful delivers a surge of important nutrients without sacrificing gourmet enjoyment.

1. 1.1 Berry Bliss Bowl

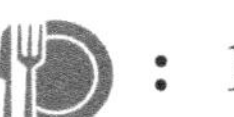 : 1   Prep  : 5 min   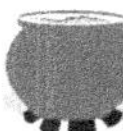 Time: 0 min

INGREDIENTS

Mixed berries (blueberries, raspberries, strawberries), spinach, almond milk, chia seeds, Greek yogurt.

DIRECTIONS

Blend berries, spinach, almond milk, chia seeds, and Greek yogurt. Top with almonds and chia seeds.

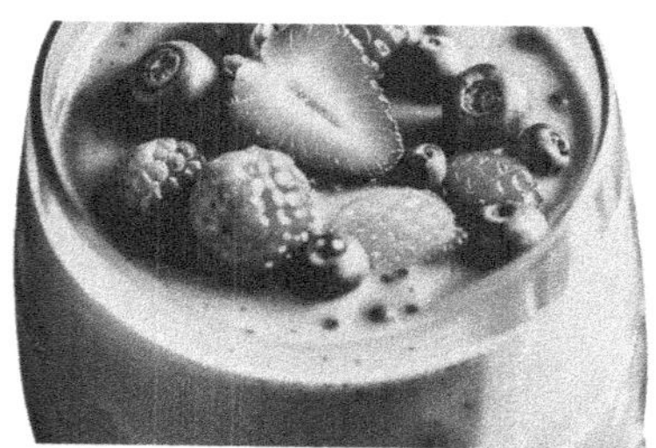

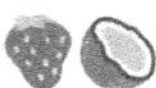

Berry Bliss Bowl: Fruity delight!

1.1.2 Green Goddess Bowl

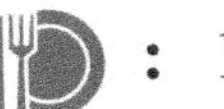 : 1   **Prep**  : 7 min   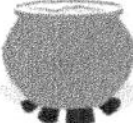 Time: 0 min

INGREDIENTS

Spinach, kale, cucumber, avocado, green apple, unsweetened coconut water.

DIRECTIONS

Blend spinach, kale, cucumber, avocado, apple, and coconut water. Top with kiwi, pumpkin seeds, and flaxseed oil.

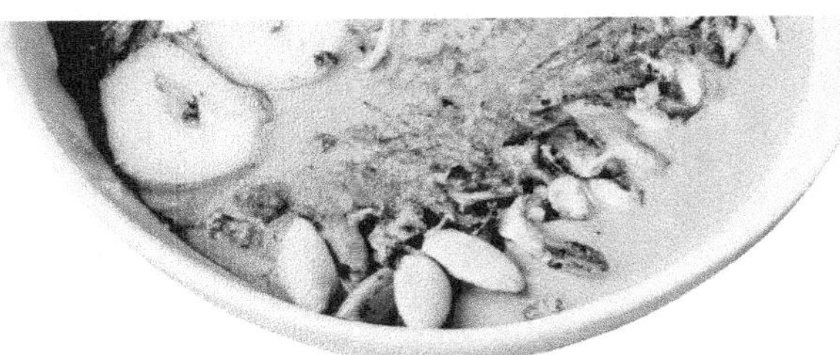

Green Goddess Bowl

1.1. 3. Protein Power Bowl

 : 1   **Prep**  : 5 min   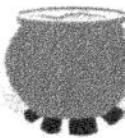 Time: 0 min

INGREDIENTS

Whey protein powder, almond butter, banana, unsweetened almond milk, spinach.

DIRECTIONS

Blend protein powder, almond butter, banana, almond milk, and spinach. Top with strawberries, hemp seeds, and Greek yogurt.

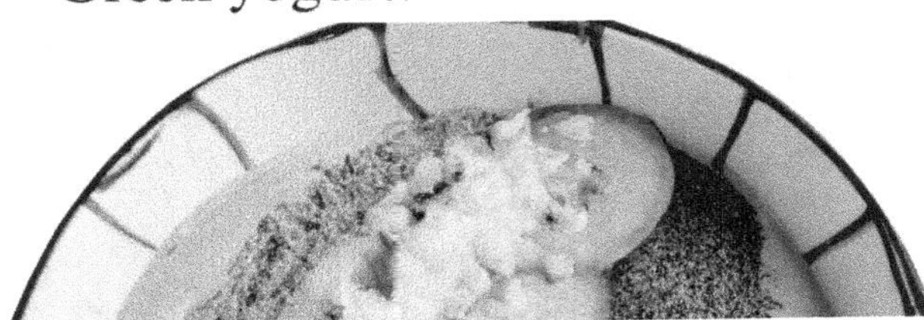

Protein Power Bowl

1.1. 4 Cinnamon Apple Delight Bowl

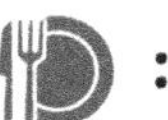 : 1　　Prep  : 6 min　　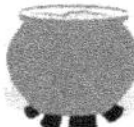 Time: 0 min

INGREDIENTS

Apple slices, cinnamon, ground flaxseeds, unsweetened soy milk, ice cubes.

DIRECTIONS

Blend apple slices, cinnamon, flaxseeds, soy milk, and ice. Top with diced apples and walnuts.

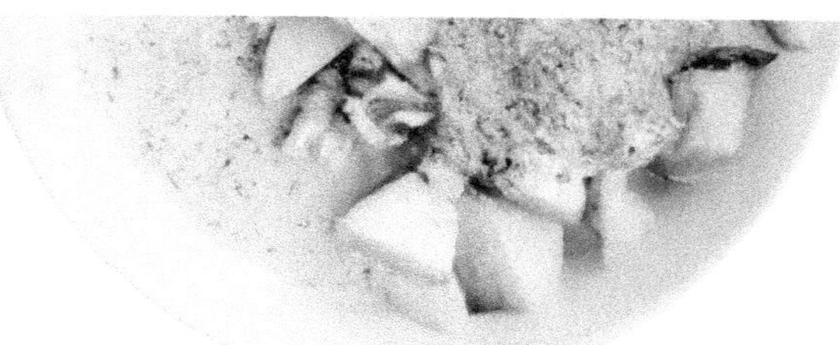

Cinnamon Apple Delight Bowl

1.1 5. Tropical Paradise Bowl

 : 1　　Prep  : 5 min　　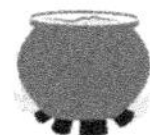 Time: 0 min

INGREDIENTS

Pineapple chunks, mango, kale, coconut water, chia seeds.

DIRECTIONS

Blend pineapple, mango, kale, coconut water, and chia seeds. Top with banana, shredded coconut, and papaya.

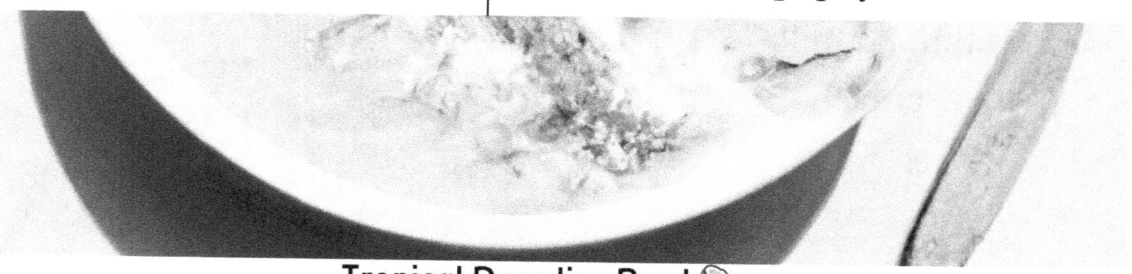

Tropical Paradise Bowl

1.1.6 Blueberry Muffin Bowl

 : 1   **Prep**  : 4 min   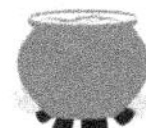 Time: 0 min

INGREDIENTS

Frozen blueberries, oats, almond milk, cinnamon, vanilla extract.

DIRECTIONS

Blend blueberries, oats, almond milk, cinnamon, and vanilla. Top with granola, fresh blueberries, and sugar-free maple syrup.

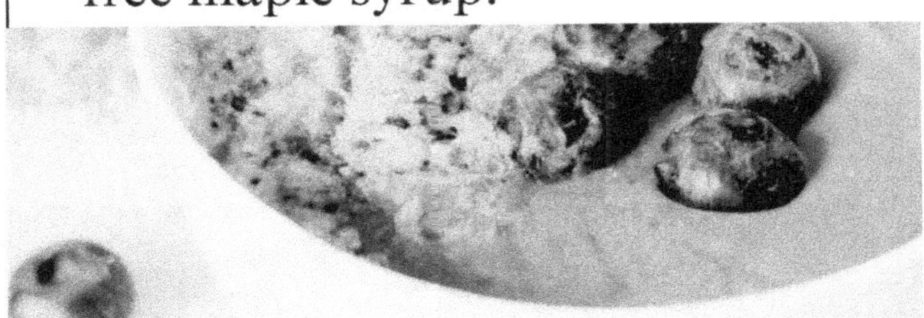

Blueberry Muffin Bowl

1.1. 7 Chocolate Peanut Butter Heaven Bowl

 : 1   **Prep**  : 6 min   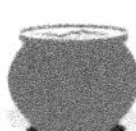 Time: 0 min

INGREDIENTS

Cocoa powder, peanut butter, banana, unsweetened almond milk, spinach.

DIRECTIONS

Blend cocoa powder, peanut butter, banana, almond milk, and spinach. Top with crushed peanuts, sliced banana, and cocoa nibs.

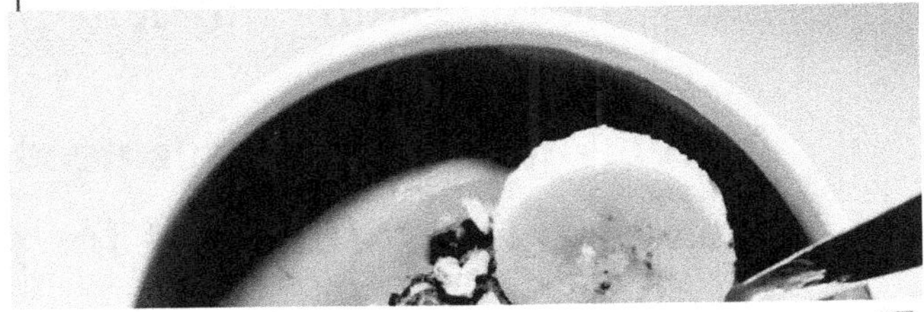

Chocolate Peanut Butter Heaven Bowl

1.1. 8 Avocado Citrus Zing Bowl

 : 1   Prep  : 6 min   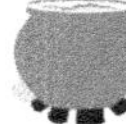 Time: 0 min

INGREDIENTS

Avocado, orange segments, banana, spinach, lime juice, almond milk.

DIRECTIONS

Blend avocado, orange segments, banana, spinach, lime juice, and almond milk until smooth. Top with sliced citrus fruits and a sprinkle of pumpkin seeds.

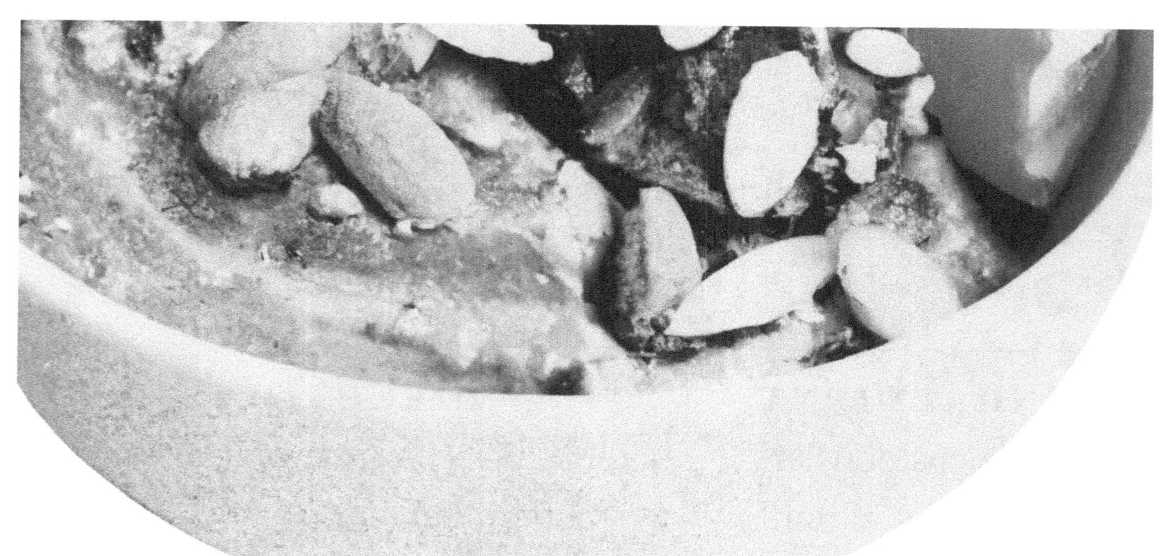

Zesty mornings: Avocado Citrus Zing Bowl. 🥑🍊

Enjoy the refreshing nutrient-packed smoothie bowls.

Note: Adjust portions as needed and consult with a healthcare professional for personalized dietary guidance.

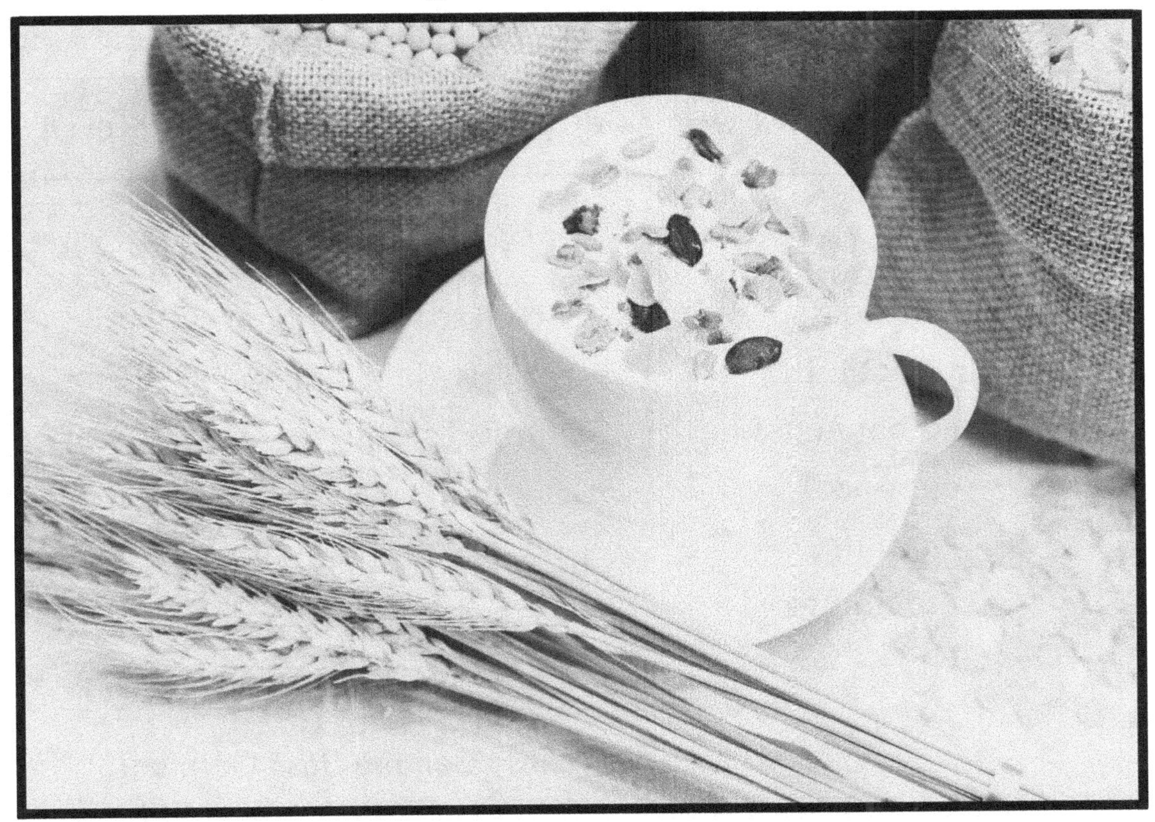

1.2 Wholesome Oatmeal Variations

When it comes to controlling Type 2 Diabetes, it is critical to prepare meals that are both nutritious and tasty. Oatmeal, with its fiber-rich and heart-healthy characteristics, serves as a fantastic canvas for producing nutritional recipes that help to maintain blood sugar levels. Join me on a gourmet adventure through Wholesome Oatmeal Variations, each meticulously crafted to balance flavor, nutrition, and diabetes-friendly ingredients.

1.2.1 Nutty Banana Bliss Oatmeal

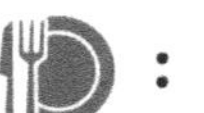 : 1   **Prep**  : 5 min   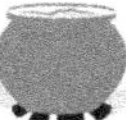 Time: 10 min

INGREDIENTS

Rolled oats, almond milk, sliced bananas, chopped walnuts, cinnamon.

DIRECTIONS

Cook oats with almond milk, top with banana slices, walnuts, and a sprinkle of cinnamon.

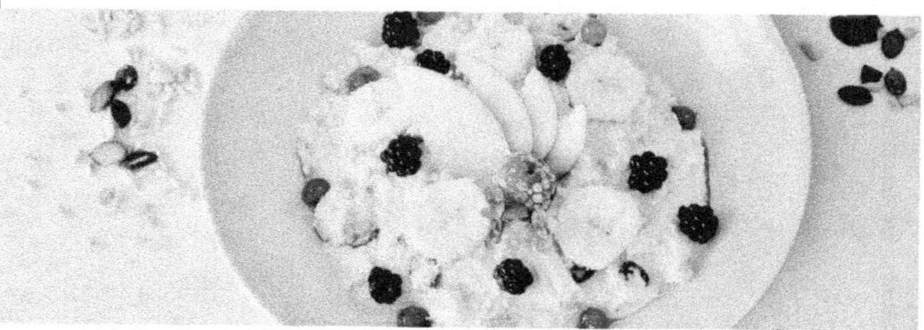

Nutty Banana Bliss Oatmeal

1.2.2. Berry Almond Delight Oatmeal

 : 1   **Prep**  : 5 min   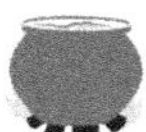 Time: 8 min

INGREDIENTS

Steel-cut oats, mixed berries, almond butter, chia seeds.

DIRECTIONS

Cook steel-cut oats, mix in berries, top with almond butter and chia seeds.

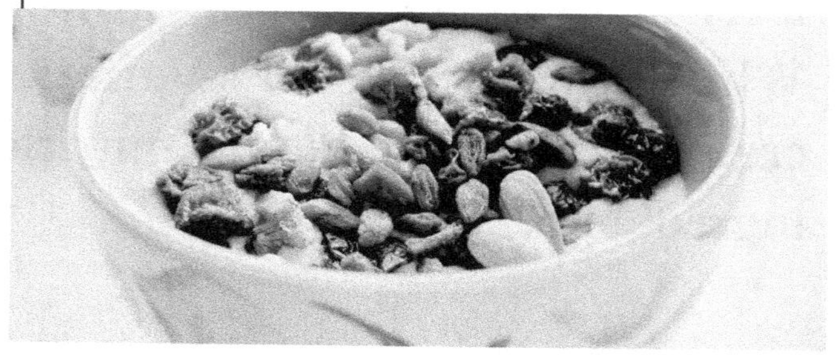

Berry Almond Oat Delight

1.2.3. Apple Cinnamon Crunch Oatmeal

 : 1  Prep : 7 min 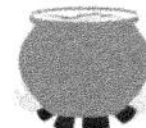 Time: 12 min

INGREDIENTS

Old-fashioned oats, diced apples, ground flaxseeds, a touch of honey.

DIRECTIONS

Cook oats with diced apples, stir in flaxseeds, and sweeten with a drizzle of honey.

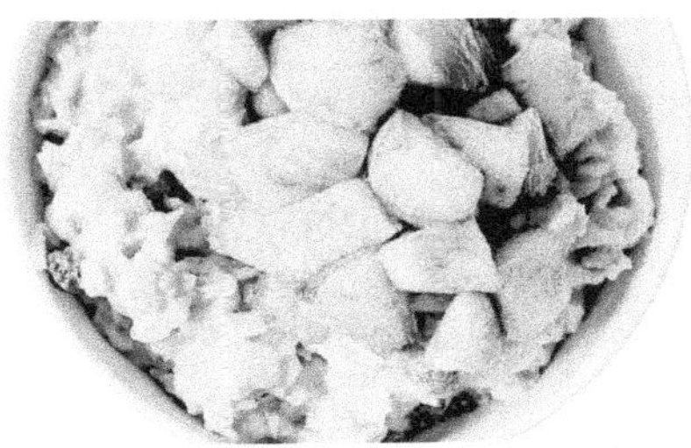

Crunchy bliss: Apple Cinnamon Oats. 

1.2.4. Tropical Coconut Crunch Oatmeal

 : 1  Prep : 5 min 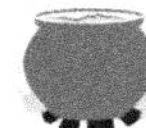 Time: 10 min

INGREDIENTS

Quick oats, coconut milk, diced mango, shredded coconut, chopped macadamia nuts.

DIRECTIONS

Cook quick oats in coconut milk, top with diced mango, shredded coconut, and chopped macadamia nuts.

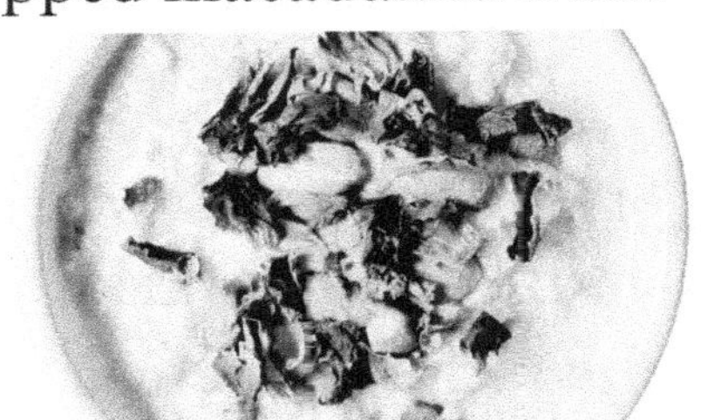

Tropical Coconut Crunch Oats 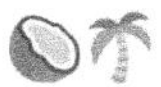

1.2.5 Pumpkin Spice Protein Oatmeal

 : 1   Prep  : 5 min   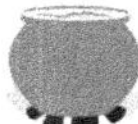 Time: 8 min

INGREDIENTS

Rolled oats, canned pumpkin puree, unsweetened almond milk, protein powder, pumpkin spice.

DIRECTIONS

Cook oats with pumpkin puree and almond milk, stir in protein powder, and sprinkle with pumpkin spice.

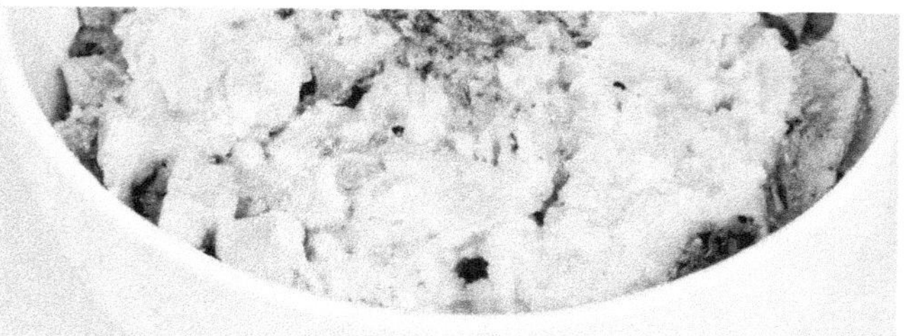

Pumpkin Spice Protein Oatmeal

1.2.6. Blueberry Lemon Burst Oatmeal

 : 1   Prep  : 6 min   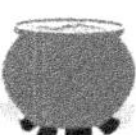 Time: 10 min

INGREDIENTS

Steel-cut oats, fresh blueberries, lemon zest, slivered almonds.

DIRECTIONS

Cook steel-cut oats, mix in fresh blueberries, sprinkle with lemon zest, and top with slivered almonds.

Note:

These oatmeal recipes prioritize diabetes-friendly nutrition. Monitor blood sugar levels, consult with your healthcare provider, and customize recipes as needed. Enjoy these wholesome variations as part of a balanced approach to managing Type 2 Diabetes.

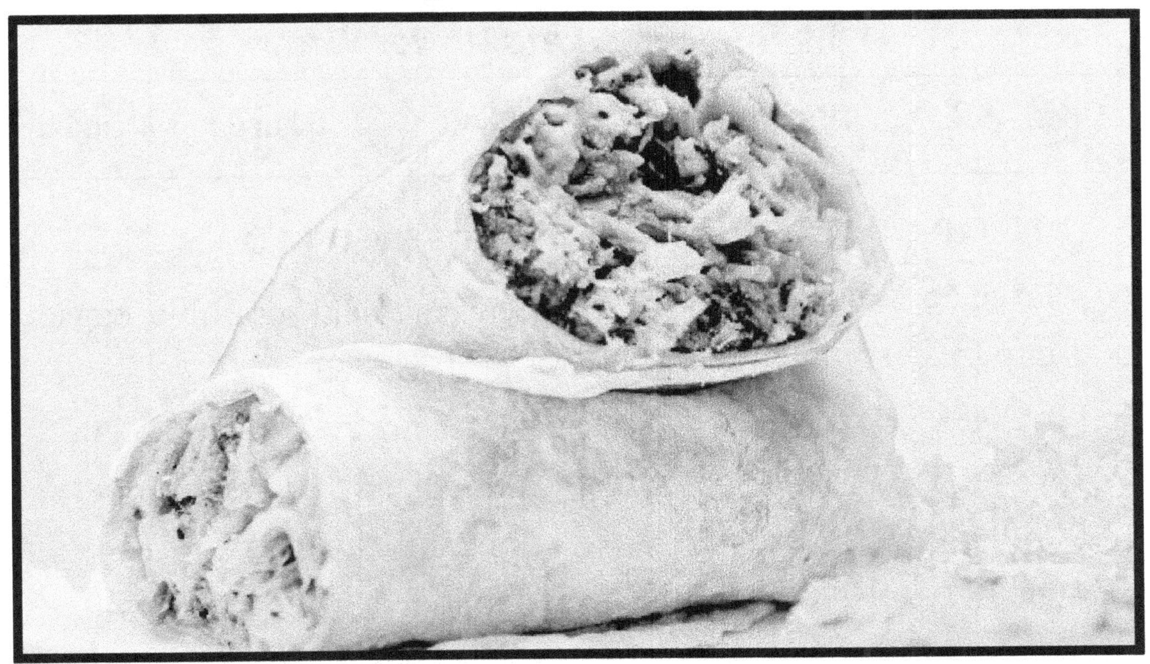

1.3 Protein-Rich Breakfast Burritos

Boost your mornings with Protein-Rich Breakfast Burritos, a savory start that blends critical nutrients with powerful tastes. These protein-packed burritos are meant to power your day while keeping you satisfied. Let's look at four hearty variants that promise to start your morning with a great protein boost.

As you go to the recipiles in the following pages Note:
Adjust portions to fit your dietary needs. These Protein-Rich Breakfast Burritos offer versatility, providing a hearty and nutritious start to your day.

1.3.1. Spinach & Feta Power Wrap

 : 2   Prep  : 10 min   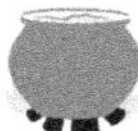 Time: 10 min

INGREDIENTS

- 4 large eggs, beaten
- 1 cup fresh spinach, chopped
- 1/2 cup feta cheese, crumbled
- 1/4 cup red bell pepper, diced
- 2 whole wheat tortillas

DIRECTIONS

1. In a skillet, scramble eggs until cooked.
2. Add chopped spinach, feta, and diced red bell pepper; stir until spinach wilts.
3. Divide the mixture between two tortillas, wrap, and serve.

1.3.2. Black Bean & Avocado Energizer

 : 2   Prep  : 8 min   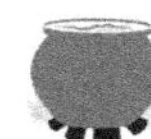 Time: 12 min

INGREDIENTS

- 1 cup black beans, canned and rinsed
- 2 large eggs, beaten
- 1/2 avocado, sliced
- 1/4 cup salsa
- 2 whole wheat tortillas

DIRECTIONS

1. Heat black beans in a skillet until warmed.
2. Scramble eggs in the same skillet until cooked.
3. Assemble burritos with black beans, scrambled eggs, avocado slices, and salsa.

1.3.3. Turkey & Veggie Protein Wrap

 : 2   Prep  : 15 min   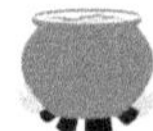 Time: 10 min

INGREDIENTS

- 1/2 lb ground turkey
- 1/2 cup bell peppers, diced
- 1/4 cup red onion, chopped
- 2 large eggs, beaten
- 2 whole wheat tortillas

DIRECTIONS

1. Brown ground turkey in a skillet, add diced peppers and chopped red onion.
2. In a separate pan, scramble eggs until done.
3. Assemble burritos with turkey mixture and scrambled eggs.

1.3.4 Veggie-Packed Breakfast Burrito

 : 2   Prep  : 12 min   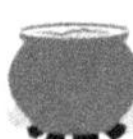 Time: 10 min

INGREDIENTS

- 1 cup mushrooms, sliced
- 1/2 cup cherry tomatoes, halved
- 1/4 cup red onion, diced
- 2 large eggs, beaten
- 2 whole wheat tortillas
- 1/4 cup shredded cheddar cheese (optional)

DIRECTIONS

1. and red onion in a skillet until tender.
2. Scramble eggs in the same skillet until cooked.
3. Divide the veggie mixture between two tortillas, add scrambled eggs, and sprinkle with shredded cheddar cheese if desired.
4. Roll up the burritos and serve.

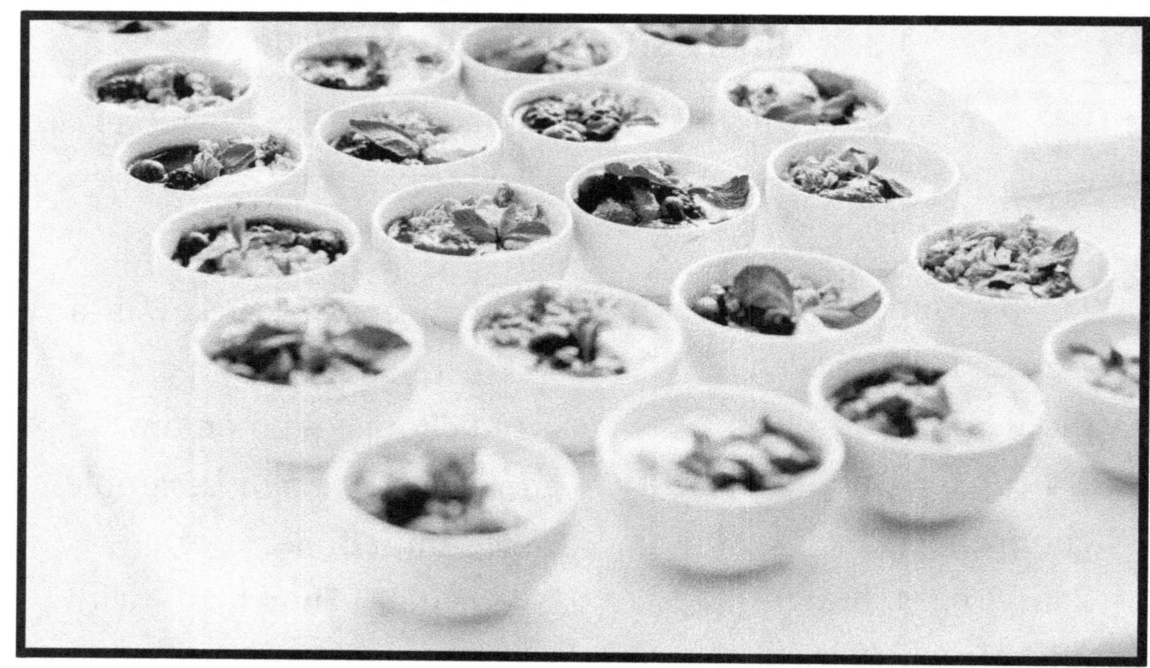

1.4 Energizing Greek Yogurt Parfaits

Rise and shine with the energizing flavor of Energizing Greek Yogurt Parfaits. These parfaits are packed with protein, probiotics, and a variety of colorful flavors, making them a delicious way to start the day. Let's look at three varieties that combine the deliciousness of Greek yogurt, fruits, and wholesome toppings to make a parfait that's both nutritious and tasty.

Feel free to customize these Energizing Greek Yogurt Parfaits to your liking. Adjust the sweetness levels, select your favorite fruits, and experiment with different toppings. These parfaits are not only a great source of energy, but they also make a tasty breakfast or snack. Enjoy the sweetness in each spoonful!

1.4.1 Berry Blast Greek Yogurt Parfait

 : 2　　　Prep 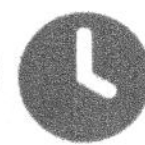 : 5 min　　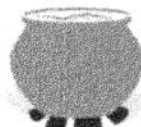 Time: 0 min

INGREDIENTS

- 1 cup Greek yogurt
- 1/2 cup mixed berries (blueberries, strawberries, raspberries)
- 2 tablespoons honey or maple syrup
- 1/4 cup granola

DIRECTIONS

1. In a glass or bowl, layer Greek yogurt, mixed berries, and drizzle with honey or maple syrup.
2. Top with a generous sprinkle of granola.
3. Repeat layers and enjoy this berry-packed delight.

1.4.2 Tropical Paradise Greek Yogurt Parfait

 : 2　　　Prep  : 6 min　　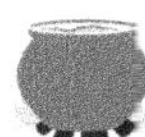 Time: 0 min

INGREDIENTS

- 1 cup Greek yogurt
- 1/2 cup pineapple chunks
- 1/2 cup mango, diced
- 2 tablespoons shredded coconut
- 1/4 cup chopped almonds

DIRECTIONS

1. Layer Greek yogurt, pineapple chunks, and diced mango in a glass or bowl.
2. Sprinkle shredded coconut and chopped almonds.
3. Repeat layers for a tropical twist in every bite.

1.4.3 Peanut Butter Banana Bliss Greek Yogurt Parfait

 : 2   Prep  : 7 min   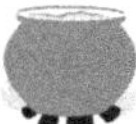 Time: 0 min

INGREDIENTS

- 1 cup Greek yogurt
- 1 banana, sliced
- 2 tablespoons peanut butter
- 1/4 cup chocolate chips (optional)

DIRECTIONS

1. In a glass or bowl, layer Greek yogurt and sliced bananas.
2. Drizzle with peanut butter and sprinkle with chocolate chips if desired.
3. Repeat layers for a decadent yet wholesome treat.

4.1.4 Cinnamon Apple Crunch Greek Yogurt Parfait

 : 2   Prep  : 8 min   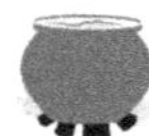 Time: 0 min

INGREDIENTS

- 1 cup Greek yogurt
- 1 apple, diced
- 2 tablespoons chopped walnuts
- 1 teaspoon cinnamon
- 1/4 cup honey or maple syrup

DIRECTIONS

1. In a glass or bowl, layer Greek yogurt and diced apples.
2. Sprinkle chopped walnuts and a dash of cinnamon.
3. Drizzle with honey or maple syrup for a sweet and spiced parfait.

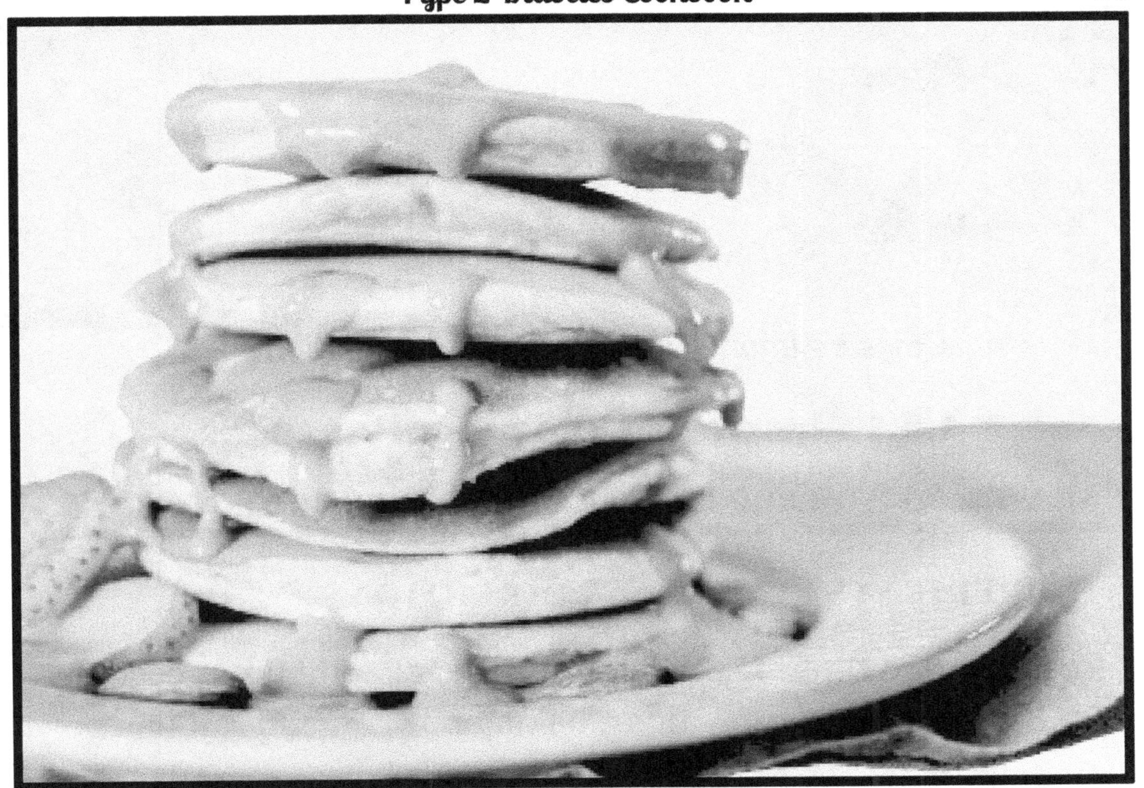

1.5 Fluffy Almond Flour Pancakes

Enjoy the amazing combination of nutty richness and gluten-free goodness with our Fluffy Almond Flour Pancakes. This recipe promises a delicious stack of pancakes that are light, fluffy, and made with healthy ingredients. Prepare to boost your breakfast experience with this delectable blend of flavor and nutrition.

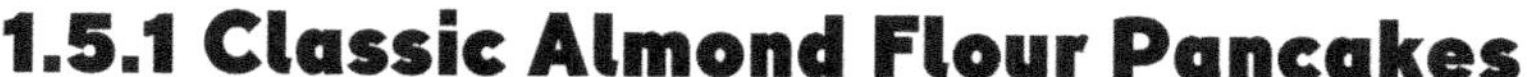

Classic Almond Pancakes: Timeless delight!

1.5.1 Classic Almond Flour Pancakes

SERVES: 2-3   PREP TIME: 10 MIN   COOK TIME: 10 MIN

INGREDIENTS

1 cup almond flour

2 tablespoons coconut flour

1 teaspoon baking powder

1/4 teaspoon salt

2 large eggs

1/2 cup almond milk

2 tablespoons melted coconut oil

1 tablespoon maple syrup

1 teaspoon vanilla extract

DIRECTIONS

1. Whisk together almond flour, coconut flour, baking powder, and salt in a bowl.
2. In a separate bowl, beat eggs, then add almond milk, melted coconut oil, maple syrup, and vanilla extract. Mix until well combined.
3. Gradually add the wet ingredients to the dry ingredients, stirring until a smooth batter forms.
4. Heat a griddle or non-stick skillet over medium heat, lightly grease with coconut oil.
5. Pour 1/4 cup of batter for each pancake onto the griddle.
6. Cook until bubbles form on the surface, then flip and cook the other side until golden brown.
7. Stack the pancakes and serve with your favorite toppings.

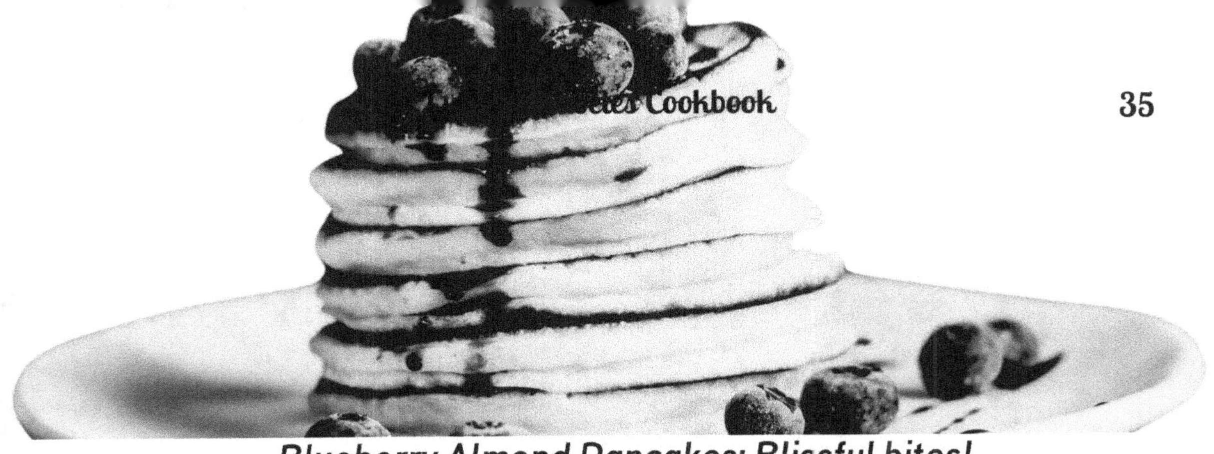

Blueberry Almond Pancakes: Blissful bites!

1.5.2 Blueberry Bliss Almond Flour Pancakes

SERVES: 2-3   **PREP TIME: 12 MIN**   **COOK TIME: 10 MIN**

INGREDIENTS

1 cup almond flour
2 tablespoons coconut flour
1 teaspoon baking powder
1/4 teaspoon salt
2 large eggs
1/2 cup almond milk
2 tablespoons melted coconut oil
1 tablespoon maple syrup
1 teaspoon vanilla extract
1/2 cup fresh blueberries

DIRECTIONS

1. Follow the same directions as for Classic Almond Flour Pancakes, adding blueberries to the batter before cooking.

Note:
Enjoy these Fluffy Almond Flour Pancakes as a delightful gluten-free option. Experiment with toppings like sliced bananas, a drizzle of honey, or a dollop of yogurt for a personalized touch. Adjust ingredients based on preferences, and relish a breakfast that combines both flavor and health.

Veggie Frittata Muffins: Bite-sized veggie goodness!

1.6 Veggie-Packed Frittata Muffins

SERVES: 4   **PREP TIME: 15 MIN**   **COOK TIME: 25 MIN**

INGREDIENTS

6 large eggs

1/2 cup diced bell peppers (assorted colors)

1/2 cup diced zucchini

1/4 cup diced red onion

1/4 cup feta cheese, crumbled

1 tablespoon olive oil

Fresh herbs (such as parsley) for garnish

DIRECTIONS

1. Preheat the oven to 375°F (190°C) and grease a muffin tin.
2. In a skillet, sauté bell peppers, zucchini, and red onion in olive oil until softened.
3. In a bowl, whisk eggs and fold in the sautéed vegetables. Spoon the mixture into muffin cups and sprinkle feta on top.
4. Bake for 20-25 minutes until the muffins are set and golden.
5. Garnish with fresh herbs before serving.

Note:

Frittata muffins – a portable, bite-sized version of a classic. Packed with colorful veggies and creamy feta, these muffins are a savory delight perfect for those on the go.

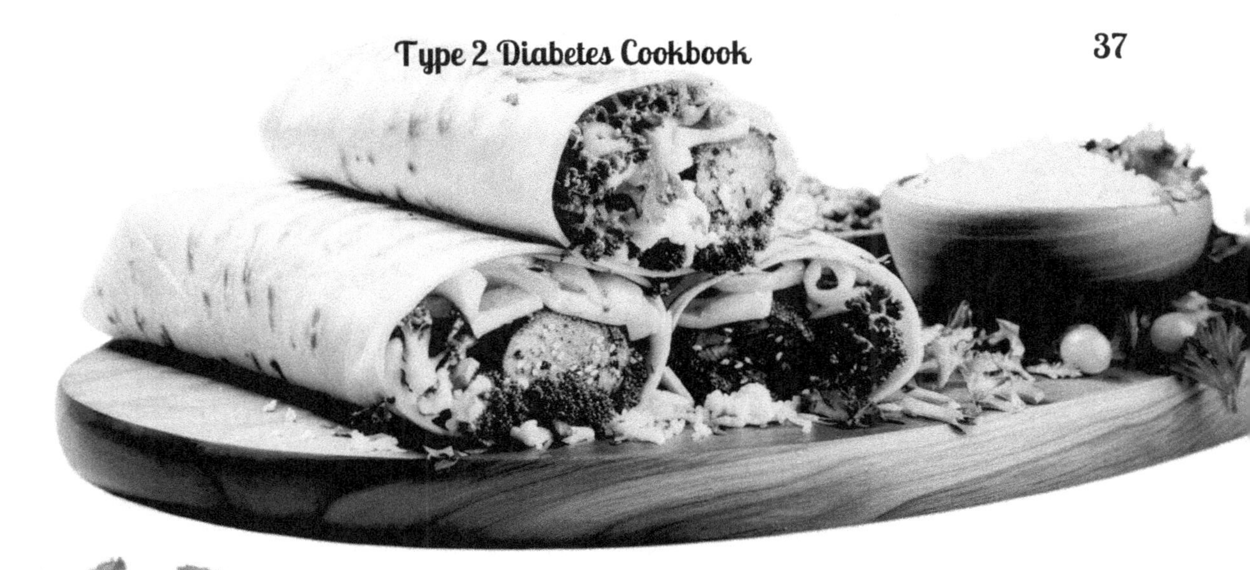

CHAPTER 2
LUNCHTIME DELIGHTS FOR DIABETES MANAGEMENT

Lunchtime is a midday break that deserves to refresh your body while also treating your taste buds. In this chapter, we'll look at a variety of lunchtime treats designed to help with diabetes management. These recipes, which range from vivid salads to protein-packed burgers, seek to make lunch not only a necessary but also an enjoyable part of your wellness journey.

Dive into a world of diabetic-friendly lunchtime treats. From grilled chicken salads to tasty soups, these ideas are designed to make your noon meal both delicious and balanced.

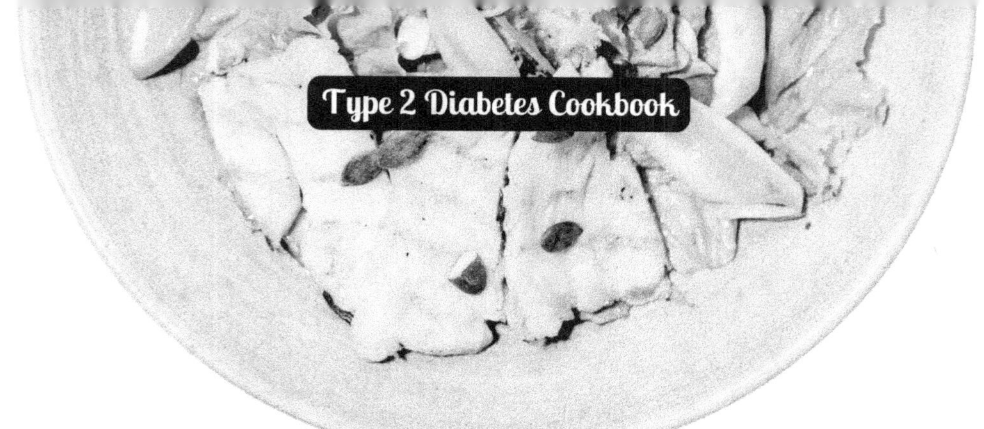

Grilled Chicken Avocado Salad: Fresh and flavorful! 🥑

2.1 Grilled Chicken Salad with Avocado Dressing

SERVES: 2   **PREP TIME: 15 MIN**   **COOK TIME: 15 MIN**

INGREDIENTS

2 boneless, skinless chicken breasts
Mixed salad greens
Cherry tomatoes, halved
Cucumber, sliced
Avocado, diced
Red onion, thinly sliced

For the dressing:
1 ripe avocado, **2** tablespoons Greek yogurt, **1** clove garlic, **2** tablespoons olive oil, **1** tablespoon lime juice, salt, and pepper to taste.

DIRECTIONS

1. Season chicken breasts with salt and pepper, then grill until cooked through.
2. In a large bowl, combine salad greens, cherry tomatoes, cucumber, diced avocado, and sliced red onion.
3. In a blender, blend all the dressing ingredients until smooth.
4. Slice grilled chicken and place it on top of the salad. Drizzle with avocado dressing.

Note:

This Grilled Chicken Salad is not just a meal; it's a symphony of textures and flavors. The creamy avocado dressing adds a delightful touch, making it a lunchtime favorite.

Quinoa & Black Bean Power Bowl: Nutrient-packed fuel!

2.2 Quinoa & Black Bean Power Bowl

SERVES: 2   **PREP TIME: 10 MIN**   **COOK TIME: 15 MIN**

INGREDIENTS

1 cup cooked quinoa
1 cup black beans, canned and rinsed
1 cup corn kernels (fresh or frozen)
1 avocado, sliced
Cherry tomatoes, halved
Fresh cilantro, chopped
Lime wedges for serving

DIRECTIONS

1. In bowls, layer cooked quinoa, black beans, corn, avocado slices, and cherry tomatoes.
2. Garnish with fresh cilantro and serve with lime wedges.

(The cooking time is for quinoa)

Note:
These Quinoa and Black Bean Power Bowls are a nutritional powerhouse. Packed with protein, fiber, and vibrant colors, they make for a satisfying lunch that keeps you energized throughout the day.

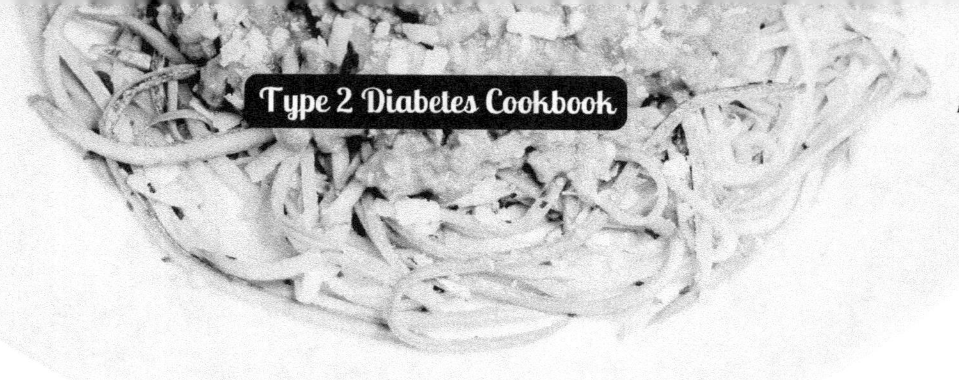

Zucchini Pesto Noodles: Fresh and flavorful! 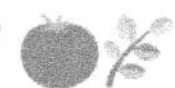

2.3 Zucchini Noodles with Pesto & Cherry Tomatoes

SERVES: 2   **PREP TIME: 15 MIN**   **COOK TIME: 0 MIN**

INGREDIENTS

3 medium zucchinis, spiralized
Cherry tomatoes, halved

For the pesto: **2** cups fresh basil, **1/2** cup pine nuts, **1/2** cup grated Parmesan cheese, **2** cloves garlic, **1/2** cup olive oil, salt, and pepper to taste.

DIRECTIONS

1. Spiralize zucchinis to create noodles.
2. In a blender, combine fresh basil, pine nuts, Parmesan cheese, garlic, and olive oil. Blend until smooth to create the pesto.
3. Toss zucchini noodles with pesto and cherry tomatoes.
4. Serve chilled.

Note:
Zucchini noodles provide a low-carb alternative in this refreshing dish. The homemade pesto adds a burst of flavor, making it a lunch option that's light on carbs but heavy on satisfaction.

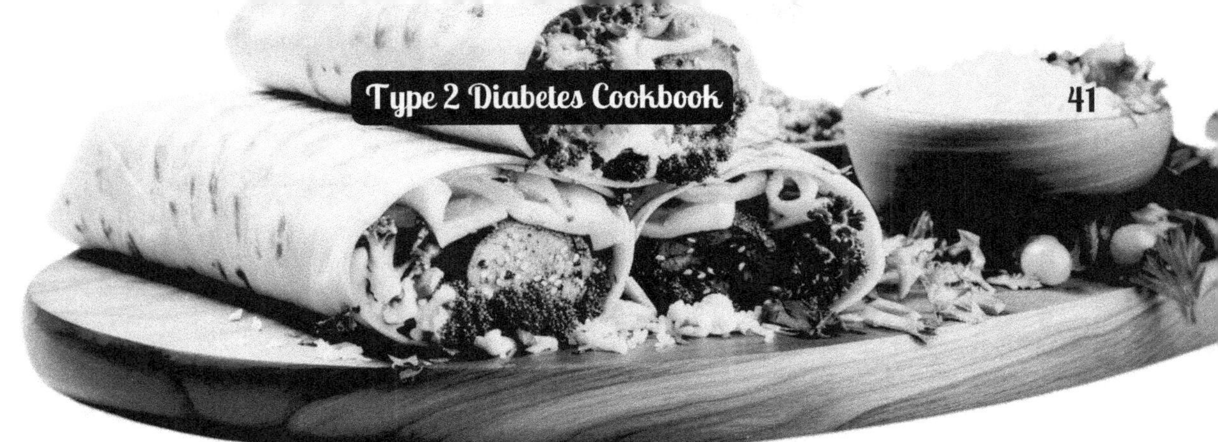

Turkey Veggie Wrap: Tasty and wholesome! 🦃

2.4 Turkey & Vegetable Wrap

SERVES: 4　　　**PREP TIME: 15 MIN**　　　**COOK TIME: 10 MIN**

INGREDIENTS

4 whole grain wraps
1/2 pound lean ground turkey
1 teaspoon olive oil
1 teaspoon cumin
1 teaspoon paprika
Salt and pepper to taste
Greek yogurt sauce:
1/2 cup Greek yogurt, 1 tablespoon lemon juice, 1 clove garlic, minced
Mixed veggies: cucumber, bell peppers, lettuce, tomatoes, thinly sliced

DIRECTIONS

1. In a skillet, heat olive oil and cook ground turkey with cumin, paprika, salt, and pepper until browned.
2. In a small bowl, mix Greek yogurt, lemon juice, and minced garlic to create the sauce.
3. Spread the Greek yogurt sauce on each wrap, add cooked turkey, and top with mixed veggies.
4. Roll the wraps and secure with toothpicks if needed.

Note:
This Turkey and Vegetable Wrap is a balanced meal in the palm of your hand. The lean turkey, fresh veggies, and zesty Greek yogurt sauce create a flavorful ensemble that's both satisfying and diabetes-friendly.

Cauli Fried Rice: Low-carb delight!

2.5 Cauliflower Fried Rice

SERVES: 2   **PREP TIME: 15 MIN**   **COOK TIME: 10 MIN**

INGREDIENTS

1 head cauliflower, grated
2 tablespoons sesame oil
1 cup mixed vegetables (peas, carrots, corn)
2 eggs, beaten
3 tablespoons low-sodium soy sauce
Green onions, chopped for garnish

DIRECTIONS

1. In a large skillet, heat sesame oil and sauté grated cauliflower and mixed vegetables until tender.
2. Push the cauliflower mixture to one side of the skillet and pour beaten eggs into the other side. Scramble the eggs until cooked.
3. Combine scrambled eggs with the cauliflower mixture. Stir in soy sauce.
4. Garnish with chopped green onions before serving.

Note:

Cauliflower Fried Rice offers all the savory satisfaction of traditional fried rice without the carb overload. It's a delicious and diabetes-friendly twist to your lunchtime routine.

Salmon Quinoa Peppers: Nutrient-packed bliss!

2.6 Salmon & Quinoa Stuffed Peppers

SERVES: 2   **PREP TIME: 15 MIN**   **COOK TIME: 25 MIN**

INGREDIENTS

2 large bell peppers, halved and seeds removed

1 cup cooked quinoa

1 can salmon, drained

1 cup cherry tomatoes, halved

1/4 cup feta cheese, crumbled

Fresh dill for garnish

DIRECTIONS

1. Preheat the oven to 375°F (190°C).
2. In a bowl, combine cooked quinoa, canned salmon, cherry tomatoes, and crumbled feta.
3. Stuff each bell pepper half with the quinoa mixture.
4. Bake for 20-25 minutes until the peppers are tender.
5. Garnish with fresh dill before serving.

Note:

The Salmon and Quinoa Stuffed Peppers are a delicious blend of flavors and textures. The quinoa and salmon combine to form a protein-rich filling, giving this a healthful and delicious lunch alternative.

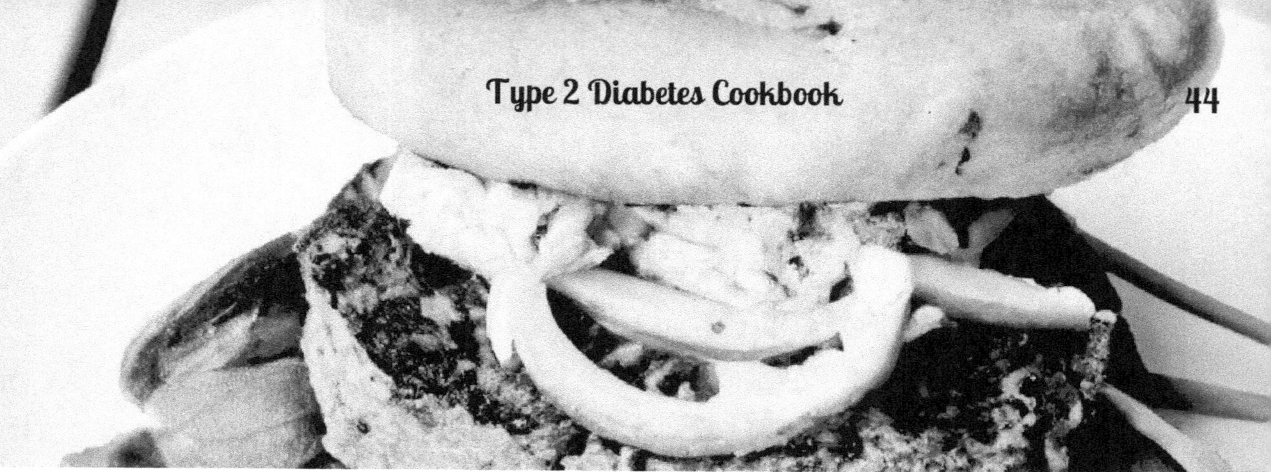

Spinach Feta Turkey Burgers: Flavor-packed! 🍔🌿

2.7 Spinach & Feta Turkey Burgers

SERVES: 4   **PREP TIME: 15 MIN**   **COOK TIME: 15 MIN**

INGREDIENTS

1 pound ground turkey

1 cup fresh spinach, chopped

1/2 cup feta cheese, crumbled

1 teaspoon dried oregano

Salt and pepper to taste

Whole grain burger buns

Toppings: lettuce, tomato slices, red onion

DIRECTIONS

1. In a bowl, mix ground turkey, chopped spinach, crumbled feta, dried oregano, salt, and pepper.
2. Form the mixture into burger patties and grill until cooked through.
3. Serve on whole grain buns with your choice of toppings.

Note:

These Spinach and Feta Turkey Burgers are a unique take on the classic, providing a lean protein source with the added benefits of spinach and feta. A lunchtime staple that is both tasty and diabetic-friendly.

Caprese Salad: Balsamic drizzle perfection! 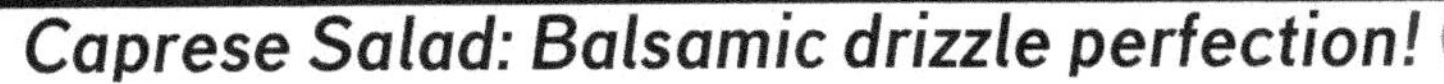

2.8 Caprese Salad with Balsamic Glaze

SERVES: 4   **PREP TIME: 10 MIN**   **COOK TIME: 0 MIN**

INGREDIENTS

4 large tomatoes, sliced

1 pound fresh mozzarella cheese, sliced

Fresh basil leaves

Balsamic glaze for drizzling

Salt and pepper to taste

DIRECTIONS

1. Arrange tomato slices and mozzarella cheese on a serving platter.
2. Tuck fresh basil leaves between tomato and mozzarella slices.
3. Drizzle with balsamic glaze and sprinkle with salt and pepper.

Note:

This Lentil and Vegetable Soup is a bowl of comfort that doesn't compromise on flavor. Packed with fiber and nutrients, it's a wholesome option for a diabetes-friendly lunch.

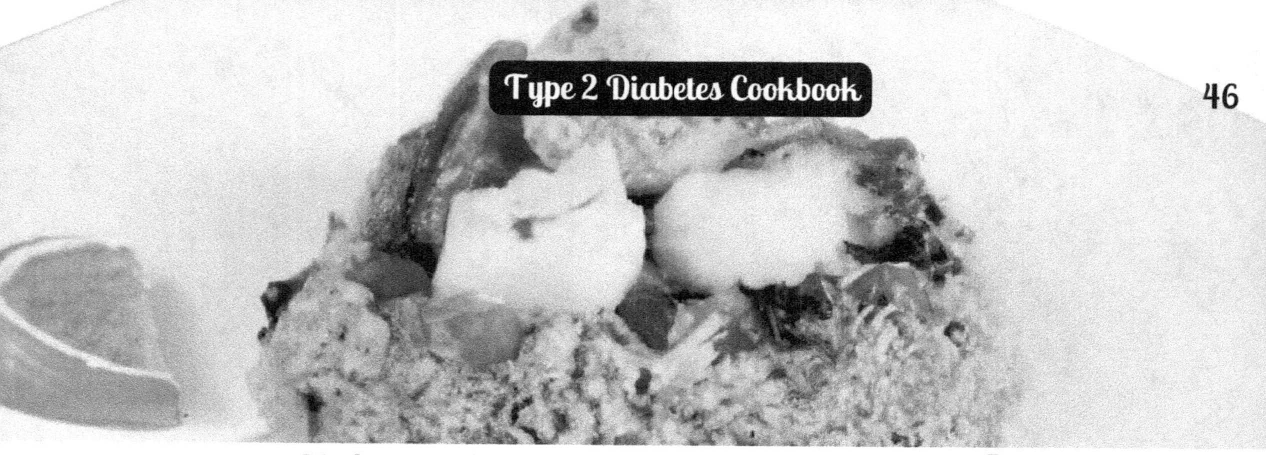

Shrimp Quinoa Salad: Light and delightful!

2.9 Shrimp & Quinoa Salad

SERVES: 2   **PREP TIME: 15 MIN**   **COOK TIME: 10 MIN**

INGREDIENTS

1 cup cooked quinoa
1 pound shrimp, peeled and deveined
1 tablespoon olive oil
1 teaspoon smoked paprika
1/2 teaspoon cayenne pepper
Mixed greens
1 cup cherry tomatoes, halved
1/4 cup feta cheese, crumbled
Lemon wedges for serving

DIRECTIONS

1. In a bowl, toss shrimp with olive oil, smoked paprika, and cayenne pepper. Grill until cooked.
2. In a large salad bowl, combine cooked quinoa, mixed greens, cherry tomatoes, and crumbled feta.
3. Top the salad with grilled shrimp and serve with lemon wedges.

Note:
This Shrimp and Quinoa Salad is a symphony of flavors. The smoky grilled shrimp paired with the lightness of quinoa and freshness of veggies create a lunch that's both satisfying and diabetes-friendly.

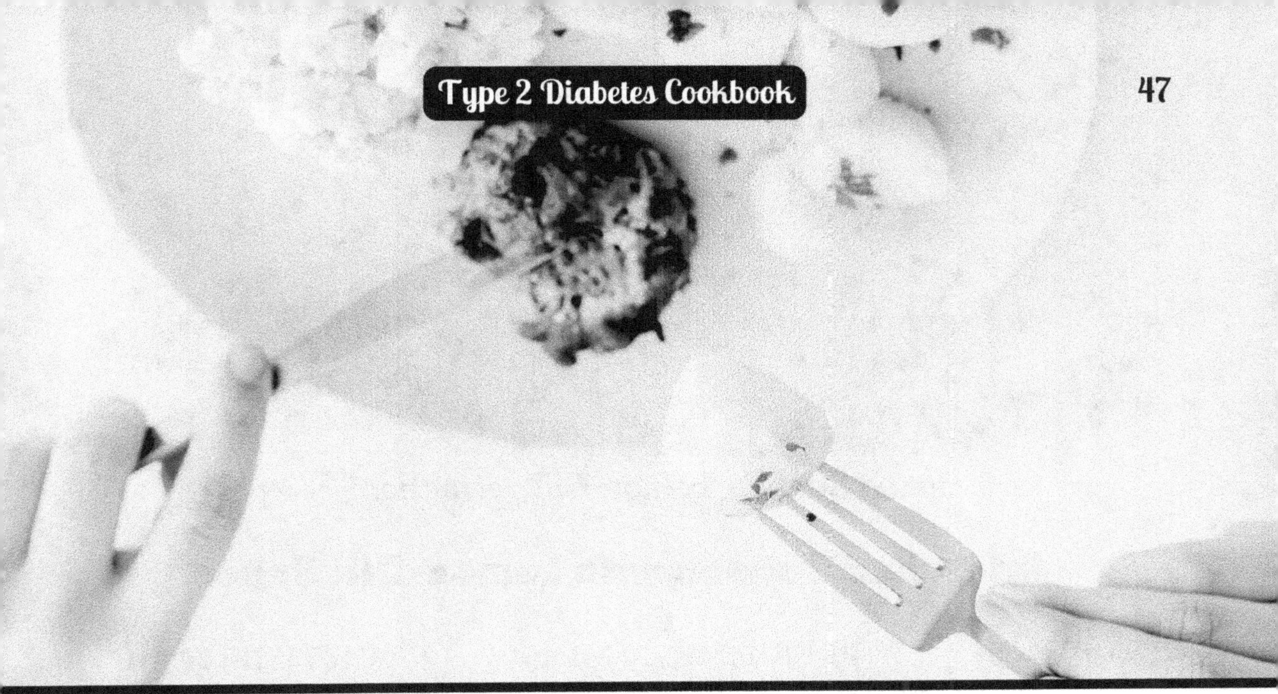

CHAPTER 3
DINNER SOLUTIONS FOR TYPE 2 DIABETES

Dinner, a time to relax and refuel, should be both satisfying and beneficial to your Type 2 Diabetes treatment. In this chapter, we look at a variety of supper options that bring delightful flavors to your table without compromising your health. From delectable baked salmon to substantial lentil stew, these dishes strive to make your meal both delicious and diabetes-friendly.

Dive into a world of meal solutions designed to help you manage Type 2 Diabetes.

Baked Salmon: Lemon-Dill perfection!

3.1 Baked Salmon with Lemon-Dill Sauce

SERVES: 2   **PREP TIME: 10 MIN**   **COOK TIME: 20 MIN**

INGREDIENTS

2 salmon fillets
1 tablespoon olive oil
1 sliced lemon
Fresh dill for garnish
Salt and pepper to taste.

DIRECTIONS

1. Preheat your oven to 375°F (190°C).
2. Arrange salmon fillets on a baking pan. Drizzle with olive oil, then season with salt and pepper.
3. Top with lemon slices and bake for 15-20 minutes, or until salmon is fully done.
4. Sprinkle with fresh dill before serving.

Note:

Baked Salmon with Lemon-Dill Sauce is an easy and delicious supper option. The tangy aromas of lemon and dill enhance the richness of salmon, resulting in a dish that is both nutritious and delicious.

Squash Bolognese: A tasty twist!

3.2 Spaghetti Squash with Turkey Bolognese

SERVES: 4   **PREP TIME: 15 MIN**   **COOK TIME: 60 MIN**

INGREDIENTS

1 medium spaghetti squash
1 pound of lean ground turkey
1 chopped onion
2 minced garlic cloves
1 can smashed tomatoes
1 teaspoon dry oregano.
1 teaspoon dried basil
Season to taste with salt and pepper Garnish with fresh parsley Top with grated Parmesan cheese.

DIRECTIONS

1. Preheat your oven to 375°F (190°C).
2. Cut the spaghetti squash in half, remove the seeds, and bake for 40 to 45 minutes.
3. In a skillet, sauté the ground turkey, onion, and garlic until browned.
4. Add the smashed tomatoes, oregano, basil, salt, and pepper to the skillet. Simmer for fifteen minutes.
5. Add spaghetti squash strands to a bowl and cover with turkey Bolognese. Garnish with fresh parsley and grated Parmigiano.

Note:
This Spaghetti Squash with Turkey Bolognese is a low-carb take on a popular dish.

Chicken Veg Stir-Fry: Quick and flavorful!

3.3 Chicken & Vegetable Stir-Fry

SERVES: 4   **PREP TIME: 20 MIN**   **COOK TIME: 15 MIN**

INGREDIENTS

1 pound boneless, skinless chicken breasts, sliced
2 cups broccoli florets
1 red bell pepper, sliced
1 carrot, julienned
1 cup snap peas
3 tablespoons low-sodium soy sauce
1 tablespoon sesame oil
1 tablespoon rice vinegar
1 teaspoon honey
2 cloves garlic, minced
1 teaspoon ginger, grated
Sesame seeds for garnish

DIRECTIONS

1. Stir-fry the chicken in a wok or big skillet until it is thoroughly done. Set aside.
2. Stir-fry broccoli, red bell pepper, carrot, and snap peas in the same skillet until crisp-tender.
3. In a small bowl, combine the soy sauce, sesame oil, rice vinegar, honey, garlic, and ginger.
4. Return the fried chicken to the skillet and pour the sauce over the stir fry. Toss until evenly coated.
5. Garnish with sesame seeds before serving.

Note:

Chicken and Vegetable Stir-Fry is a quick and colorful meal alternative.

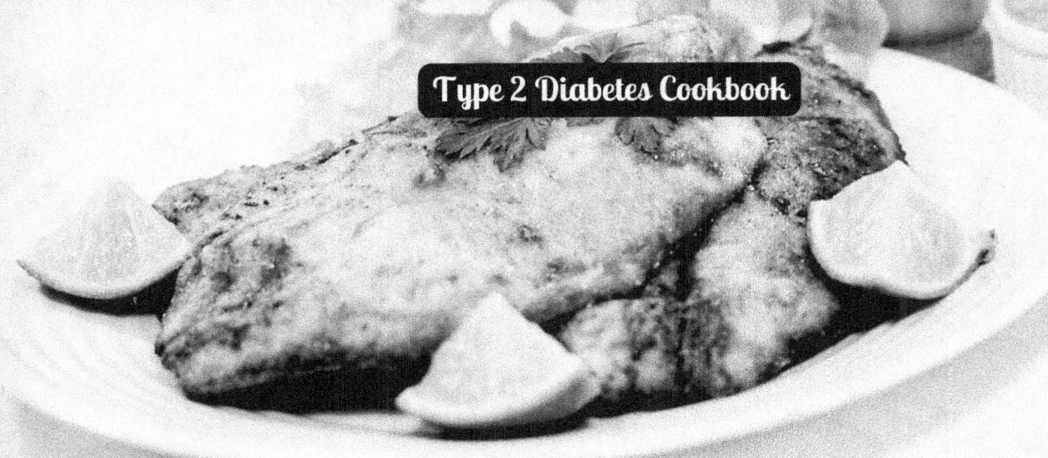

Herb-Crusted Tilapia: Flavorful perfection!

3.4 Herb-Crusted Tilapia

SERVES: 4   **PREP TIME: 10 MIN**   **COOK TIME: 15 MIN**

INGREDIENTS

4 tilapia fillets
1/2 cup almond meal
2 tablespoons fresh parsley, chopped
1 teaspoon dried thyme
1 teaspoon paprika
1 lemon, cut into wedges
Olive oil for drizzling
Salt and pepper to taste

DIRECTIONS

1. Preheat your oven to 400°F (200°C).
2. In a bowl, combine almond meal, chopped parsley, thyme, paprika, salt, and pepper.
3. Press each tilapia fillet into the herb mixture to coat both sides.
4. Place the fillets on a baking pan, spray with olive oil, and bake for 12-15 minutes, or until the fish is flaky.
5. Serve with lemon wedges.

Note:
Herb-Crusted Tilapia is a light and tasty dinner alternative. The almond meal crust provides a nutty bite, making this dish both tasty and diabetic-friendly.

Lentil Veg Stew: Hearty & wholesome!

3.5 Lentil & Vegetable Stew

SERVES: 6   **PREP TIME: 15 MIN**   **COOK TIME: 30 MIN**

INGREDIENTS

1 cup dry green lentils, rinsed
1 onion, diced
2 carrots, diced
2 celery stalks, diced
3 cloves garlic, minced
1 can diced tomatoes
6 cups vegetable broth
1 teaspoon cumin
1 teaspoon paprika
Salt and pepper to taste
Fresh parsley for garnish

DIRECTIONS

1. In a large pot, sauté the onion, carrots, celery, and garlic until tender.
2. Combine the lentils, diced tomatoes, vegetable broth, cumin, paprika, salt, and pepper. Bring to a boil.
3. Reduce the heat to a simmer for 25-30 minutes, or until the lentils are cooked.
4. Sprinkle with fresh parsley before serving.

Note:
This Lentil and Vegetable Stew provides comfort without sacrificing flavor. It's a nutritious option for a diabetes-friendly dinner.

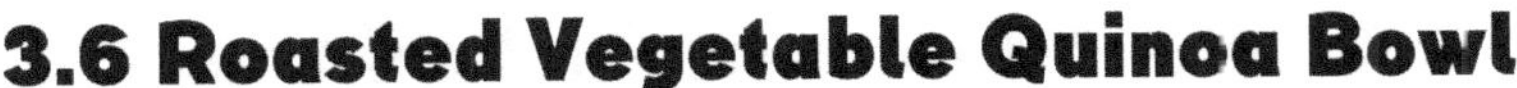

Roasted Veg Quinoa Bowl: Nutrient-packed goodness!

3.6 Roasted Vegetable Quinoa Bowl

SERVES: 2   **PREP TIME: 15 MIN**   **COOK TIME: 25 MIN**

INGREDIENTS

1 cup cooked quinoa
2 cups mixed vegetables (bell peppers, zucchini, cherry tomatoes)
1 tablespoon olive oil
1 teaspoon dried Italian herbs
Salt and pepper to taste
Feta cheese for garnish
Balsamic glaze for drizzling

DIRECTIONS

1. Pre-heat the oven to 425°F (220°C).
2. Toss the mixed veggies with olive oil, dried Italian herbs, salt, and pepper. Roast for 20-25 minutes, until the vegetables have caramelized.
3. In bowls, combine cooked quinoa and roasted vegetables.
4. Garnish with crumbled feta and drizzle with balsamic glaze.

Note:
The Roasted Vegetable Quinoa Bowl features a variety of flavors and textures. The caramelized vegetables, combined with quinoa, make for a nutritious and diabetes-friendly supper.

Citrus Chicken: Grilled perfection!

3.7 Citrus-Marinated Grilled Chicken

SERVES: 4   **PREP TIME: 10 MIN**   **COOK TIME: 15 MIN**

INGREDIENTS

4 boneless, skinless chicken breasts
1/4 cup orange juice
1/4 cup lime juice
2 tablespoons olive oil
1 teaspoon honey
2 cloves garlic, minced
1 teaspoon cumin
Salt and pepper to taste
Fresh cilantro for garnish

DIRECTIONS

1. In a bowl, combine orange juice, lime juice, olive oil, honey, minced garlic, cumin, salt, and pepper.
2. Marinate the chicken breasts in the citrus mixture for at least 30 minutes.
3. Grill the chicken until cooked through, basting with the marinade.
4. Before serving, garnish with chopped fresh cilantro.

Note:
Citrus-Marinated Grilled Chicken brings a burst of freshness to your dinner dish. The zesty marinade infuses the chicken with flavor, resulting in a dish that is both colorful and diabetic friendly.

Cauli-Broccoli Alfredo: Creamy goodness!

3.8 Cauliflower & Broccoli Alfredo

SERVES: 4   **PREP TIME: 15 MIN**   **COOK TIME: 20 MIN**

INGREDIENTS

2 cups cauliflower florets
2 cups broccoli florets
2 tablespoons olive oil
3 cloves garlic, minced
1 cup vegetable broth
1 cup unsweetened almond milk
1/4 cup nutritional yeast
Salt and pepper to taste
8 oz whole wheat fettuccine
Fresh parsley for garnish

DIRECTIONS

1. Steam the cauliflower and broccoli until they are soft.
2. In a skillet, sauté minced garlic in olive oil until aromatic.
3. Blend together steamed cauliflower, broccoli, sautéed garlic, vegetable broth, almond milk, nutritional yeast, salt, and pepper. Blend until completely smooth.
4. Cook whole wheat fettuccine according to the package directions. Drain and stir with Alfredo sauce for cauliflower and broccoli.
5. Just before serving, garnish with fresh parsley.

Note:
Cauliflower and Broccoli Alfredo is a creamy, guilt-free alternative to typical Alfredo sauce.

Eggplant Chickpea Curry: Spicy delight!

3.9 Eggplant & Chickpea Curry

SERVES: 4   **PREP TIME: 15 MIN**   **COOK TIME: 25 MIN**

INGREDIENTS

1 big eggplant, chopped

1 can chickpeas, drained and rinsed.

1 one onion, diced

3 cloves of minced garlic

1 can of chopped tomatoes

1 can coconut milk.

2 Tbsp curry powder

1 teaspoon of cumin.

1 teaspoon Turmeric

Salt & pepper to taste.

Fresh cilantro as a garnish.

Cooked brown rice ready for serving

DIRECTIONS

1. In a large pot, cook diced eggplant, onion, and garlic until softened.
2. Mix in chickpeas, chopped tomatoes, coconut milk, curry powder, cumin, turmeric, salt, and pepper. Simmer for 20 to 25 minutes.
3. Serve over cooked brown rice and sprinkle with fresh cilantro.

Note: Eggplant and Chickpea Curry is both comforting and flavorful. The combination of spices, creamy coconut milk, and substantial chickpeas makes for a delicious and diabetic-friendly meal.

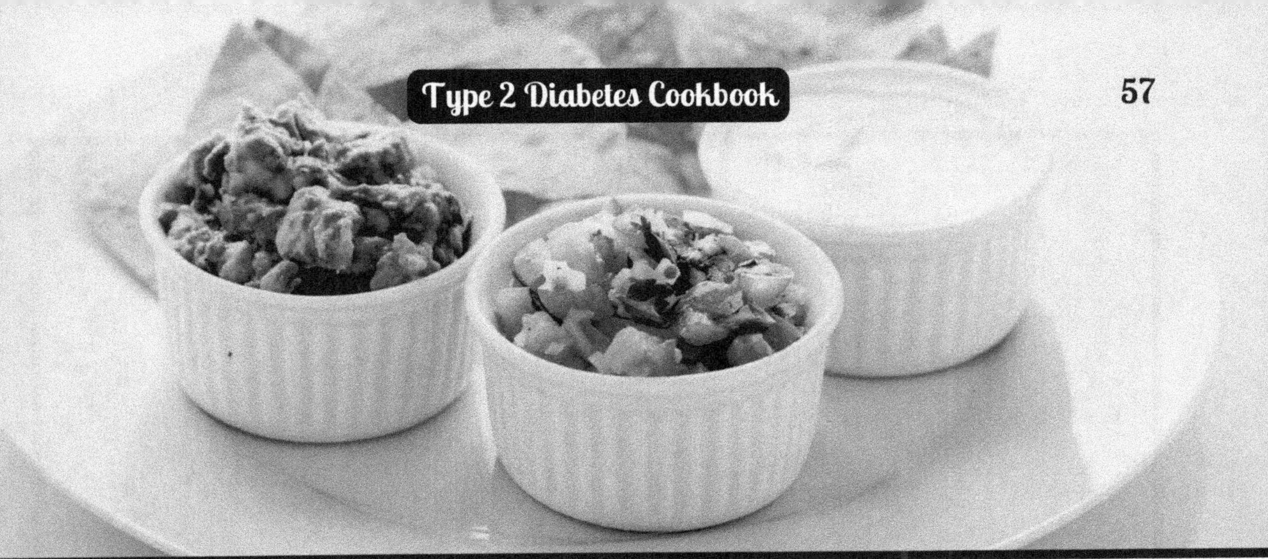

CHAPTER 4
SNACK SMART WITH TYPE 2 DIABETES-FRIENDLY BITES

Snacking can be challenging when managing Type 2 Diabetes, but it doesn't have to be bland or boring. In this chapter, we'll look at a selection of snacks that are both delicious and diabetic-friendly. These smart snacks, which range from energy-packed almond bits to refreshing Greek Yogurt Popsicles, are meant to keep you energized and your blood sugar stable.

With these diabetes-friendly bites, you can embark on a journey of smart eating. Whether you're seeking something sweet, savory, or crunchy, these snacks will keep your blood sugar stable while delighting your taste buds.

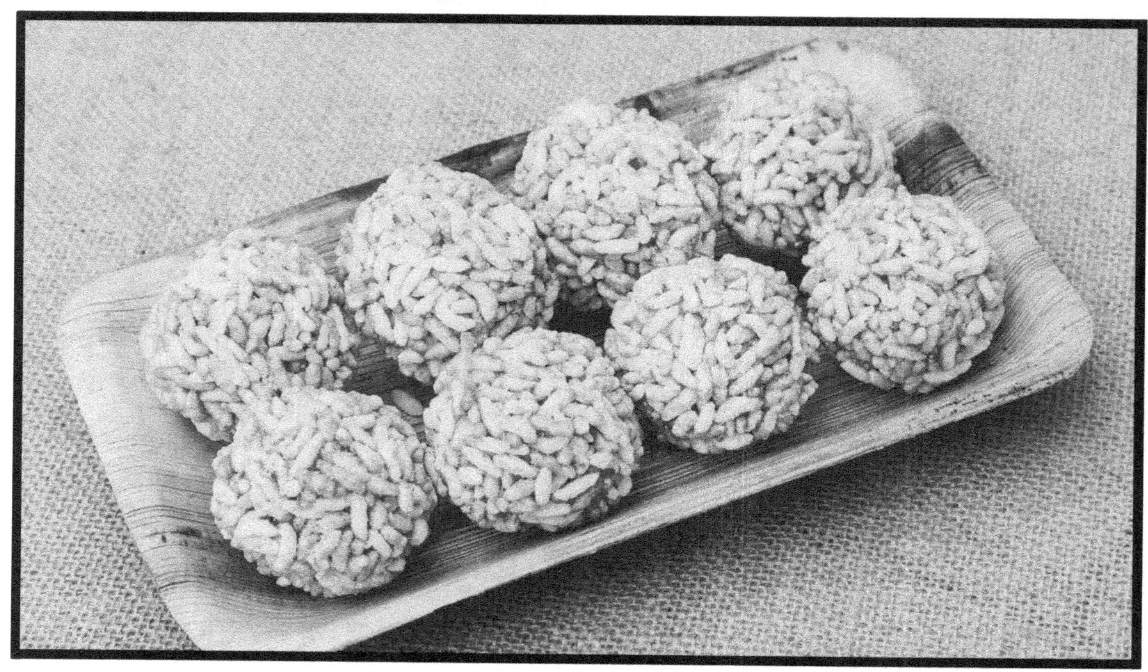

4.1 Almond and Berry Energy Bites

Almond and Berry Energy Bites are bite-sized bursts of energy and flavor. These no-bake snacks are not only delicious, but also packed with nutritious components to keep you going all day. Let's try two delicious variants that combine the nuttiness of almonds with the sweetness of berries.

These Almond and Berry Energy Bites are adaptable and may be tailored to your taste preferences. Keep them refrigerated for a fast and nutritious snack on the road. Adjust the ingredients to your preference, and eat these nutritious nibbles whenever you need a boost of energy.

4.1.1 Almond Joy Energy Bites

Yield: 12-15 bites   **Prep 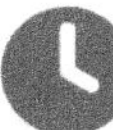 : 15 min**

INGREDIENTS

1 cup rolled oats

1/2 cup almond butter

1/4 cup honey

1/2 cup chopped almonds

1/4 cup shredded coconut

1/4 cup dark chocolate chips

1 teaspoon vanilla extract

DIRECTIONS

1. Mix oats, almond butter, honey, almonds, coconut, chocolate chips, and vanilla.
2. Roll into bite-sized balls.
3. Refrigerate for at least 30 minutes before serving.

4.1.2 Berry Almond Bliss Energy Bites

Yield: 12-15 bites   **Prep  : 15 min**

INGREDIENTS

1 cup dried mixed berries

1/2 cup almond butter

1/4 cup honey

1/2 cup almond meal

1/4 cup chopped almonds

1/4 cup chia seeds

1 teaspoon vanilla extract

DIRECTIONS

1. Pulse dried berries in a food processor.
2. Mix berries, almond butter, honey, almond meal, almonds, chia seeds, and vanilla.
3. Roll into bite-sized balls.
4. Refrigerate for at least 30 minutes before serving.

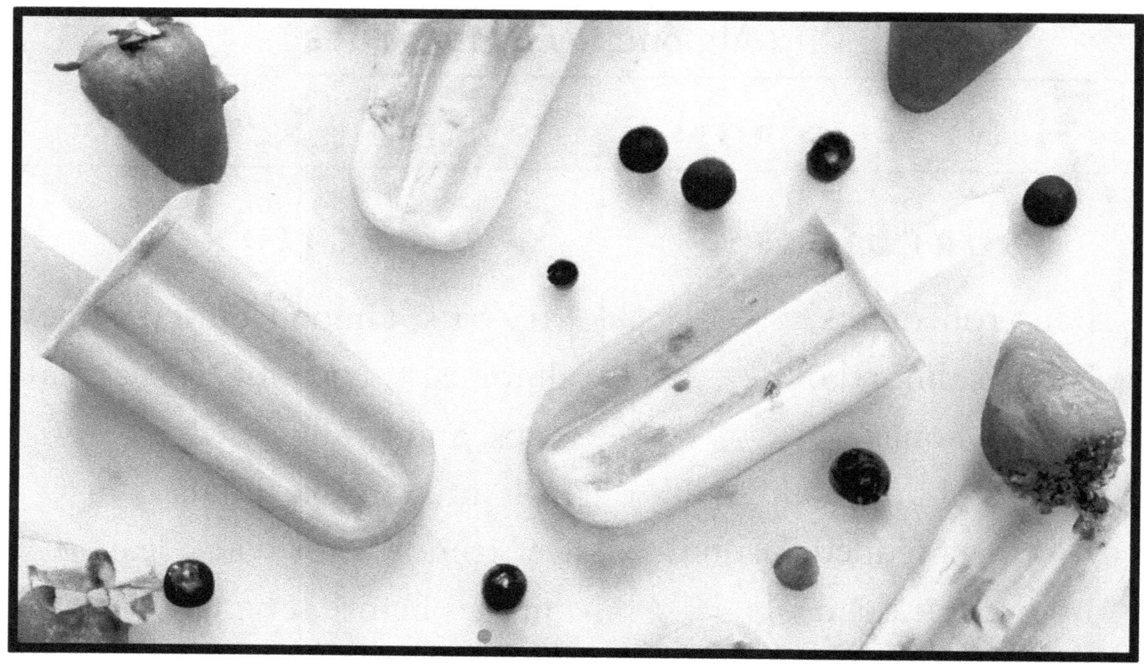

4.2 Greek Yogurt & Berry Popsicles

Greek Yogurt and Berry Popsicles are a delicious and healthful treat. These frozen treats mix the creamy deliciousness of Greek yogurt with the vivid sweetness of berries, resulting in an ideal combination of flavor and nutrition. Let's look at two simple recipes for guilt-free treats on a stick.

Enjoy these Greek Yogurt and Berry Popsicles as a tasty and healthful frozen treat. Try different berries or add a sprinkling of oats for added crunch. Be creative and enjoy the refreshing, pleasing flavor of these handmade popsicles.

4.2.1 Mixed Berry Swirl Popsicles

Yield: 6 Popsicles   **Prep  : 10 min**

INGREDIENTS

1 cup of Greek yogurt.
1/2 cup mixed berries
(strawberries, blueberries,
raspberries)
2 tablespoons honey
1 teaspoon vanilla essence.

DIRECTIONS

1. In a blender, combine the Greek yogurt, mixed berries, honey, and vanilla extract.
2. Blend until smooth.
3. Pour the mixture into popsicle molds, and top with more whole berries if desired.
4. Insert the popsicle sticks and freeze until set.

4.2.2. Blueberry Lemonade Yogurt Popsicles

Yield: 6 Popsicles   **Prep  : 10 min**

INGREDIENTS

1 cup of Greek yogurt.
1/2 cup blueberries
2 tablespoons honey
1/4 cup lemonade (freshly
squeezed or store-bought).
Zest from one lemon

DIRECTIONS

1. In a blender, combine the Greek yogurt, blueberries, honey, lemonade, and lemon zest until smooth.
2. Pour the mixture into the popsicle molds.
3. Freeze until partially firm, then insert the popsicle sticks.
4. Freeze until solid.

4.3 Veggie Sticks & Hummus

 : 2   Prep  : 10 min   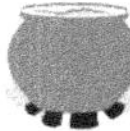 Time: 0 min

INGREDIENTS

Carrot sticks, cucumber sticks, bell pepper strips, and cherry tomatoes.
- Hummus for dipping

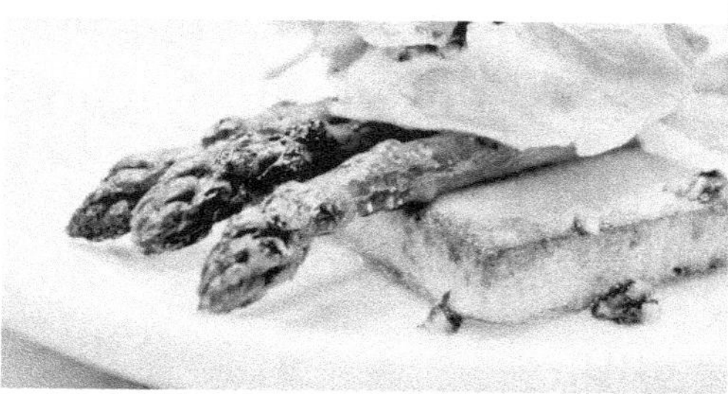

DIRECTIONS

Wash and cut the vegetables into sticks and strips.

Arrange the vegetable sticks on a platter.

Serve with a side of hummus to dip.

Note:
Veggie Sticks with Hummus are a crunchy and tasty snack.

4.4 Nutty Trail Mix

 : 4   Prep  : 5 min   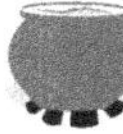 Time: 0 min

INGREDIENTS

1 cup mixed nuts (almonds, walnuts, pistachios) and 1/2 cup chopped dried apricots.
1/2 cup dark chocolate chips,
1/4 cup pumpkin seeds
1/4 teaspoon sea salt

DIRECTIONS

In a dish, combine the mixed nuts, chopped dried apricots, dark chocolate chips, pumpkin seeds, and sea salt.

Divide into snack-sized bags for easy portability.

Note:
Nutty Trail Mix is a handy and filling snack.

4.5 Quick Avocado Salsa

 : 4   Prep  : 10 min   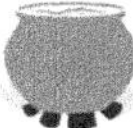 Time: 0 min

INGREDIENTS

Dice 2 ripe avocados and 1 cup cherry tomatoes.

Add 1/4 cup finely chopped red onion, 1/4 cup chopped fresh cilantro.

Juice 1 lime, then add salt and pepper to taste.

DIRECTIONS

Mix avocados, tomatoes, red onion, cilantro, lime juice, salt, and pepper in a dish.

Serve with whole-grain tortilla chips.

Note:
This Avocado and Tomato Salsa with Whole Grain Chips offers a vibrant and flavorful snack.

4.6 Cucumber & Tuna Bites

 : 4   Prep  : 10 min   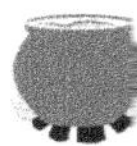 Time: 0 min

INGREDIENTS

1 cucumber sliced into rounds.

1 canned tuna, drained

Two tablespoons of Greek yogurt

1 tbsp Dijon mustard

Fresh dill as garnish

DIRECTIONS

In a bowl, combine tuna, Greek yogurt, and Dijon mustard.

Spoon the tuna mixture onto the cucumber slices.

Garnish with fresh dill and serve.

Note:
Cucumber and Tuna Bites are a light, protein-rich snack.

4.7 Apples & Almond Butter Sandwich

 : 2   Prep  : 5 min   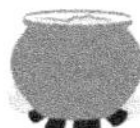 Time: 0 min

INGREDIENTS

2 apples, cored and cut into rounds.
Almond Butter
Granola for topping.

DIRECTIONS

1. Spread almond butter on one side of each apple slice.
2. Add another apple slice to make a sandwich.
3. To add crunch, dip the sandwich's edges into granola.

Note:
Apple and almond butter sandwiches are a tasty and satisfying snack.

4. 8 Spicy Roasted Chickpea

 : 4   Prep  : 10 min   Roast Time: 25 min

INGREDIENTS

2 cans drained and rinsed chickpeas
2 tablespoons olive oil
1 teaspoon ground cumin
1/2 teaspoon smoked paprika.
1/2 teaspoon garlic powder
Add salt to taste.

DIRECTIONS

1. Preheat your oven to 400°F (200°C).
2. In a bowl, combine chickpeas, olive oil, ground cumin, smoked paprika, garlic powder, and salt.
3. Spread the chickpeas on a baking sheet and roast for 20-25 minutes, until crispy.

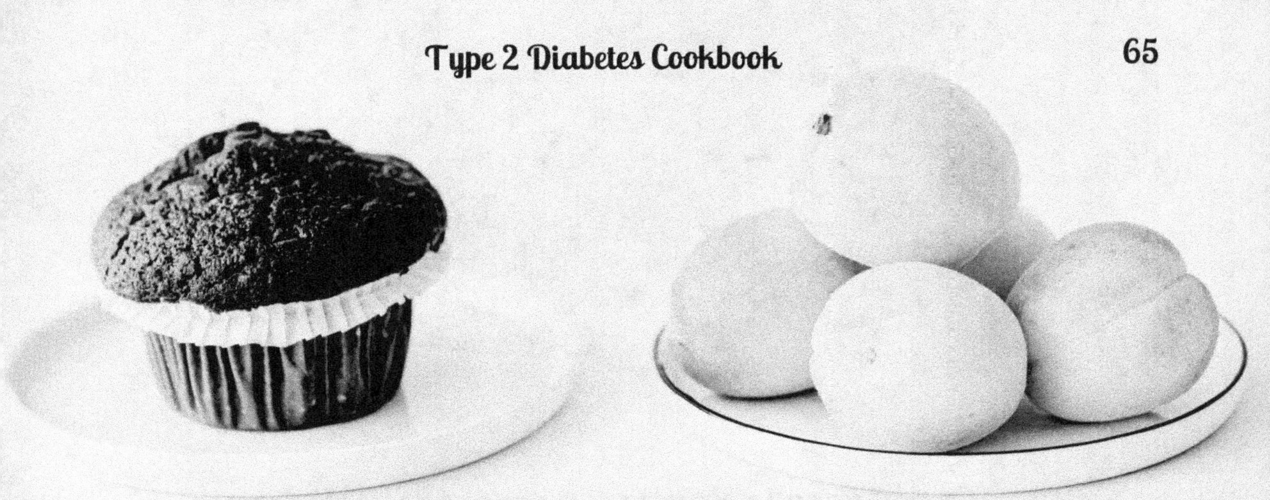

CHAPTER 5
DESSERT DELIGHTS FOR DIABETICS

Desserts need not be a forbidden indulgence for those managing Type 2 Diabetes. In this chapter, we delve into a world of sweet treats crafted specifically for individuals watching their blood sugar levels. From the richness of Dark Chocolate Avocado Mousse to the warmth of Sugar-Free Pumpkin Pie, these desserts promise to satisfy your sweet tooth without compromising your health.

Indulge your sweet cravings with these diabetes-friendly dessert options.

Choc Avocado Mousse: Decadent delight!

5.1 Dark Chocolate Avocado Mousse

SERVES: 4   **PREP TIME: 10 MIN**   **COOK TIME: 2 HRS**

INGREDIENTS

2 ripe avocados
1/2 cup unsweetened cocoa powder
1/4 cup almond milk
1/4 cup maple syrup or sugar substitute
1 teaspoon vanilla extract
Pinch of salt
Fresh berries for garnish

DIRECTIONS

1. In a blender, combine avocados, cocoa powder, almond milk, maple syrup, vanilla extract, and salt. Blend until smooth.
2. Spoon the mousse into serving glasses and refrigerate for at least 2 hours.
3. Garnish with fresh berries before serving.

Note:

Dark Chocolate Avocado Mousse is a decadent and creamy dessert that hides a nutritious secret. Avocado adds richness and a velvety texture, making this mousse a guilt-free delight.

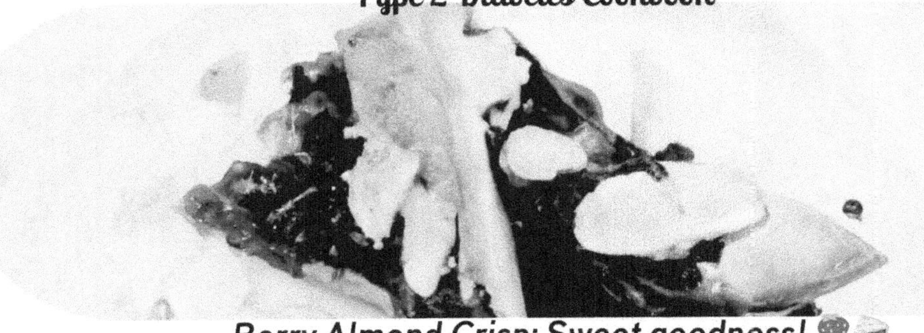

Berry Almond Crisp: Sweet goodness! 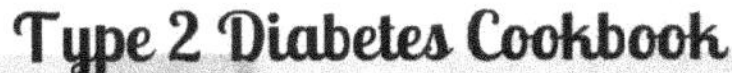

5.2 Berry & Almond Crisp

SERVES: 4   **PREP TIME: 15 MIN**   **COOK TIME: 30 MIN**

INGREDIENTS

2 cups mixed berries
(strawberries,
blueberries,
raspberries)
1 tablespoon lemon
juice
1/4 cup almond flour
1/4 cup rolled oats
2 tablespoons
chopped almonds
2 tablespoons
coconut oil, melted
2 tablespoons maple
syrup or sugar
substitute
Pinch of cinnamon
Greek yogurt for
serving

DIRECTIONS

1. Preheat the oven to 375°F (190°C).
2. In a bowl, toss mixed berries with lemon juice and spread in a baking dish.
3. In another bowl, combine almond flour, rolled oats, chopped almonds, melted coconut oil, maple syrup, and cinnamon.
4. Sprinkle the almond-oat mixture over the berries.
5. Bake for 25-30 minutes until the topping is golden and the berries are bubbly.
6. Serve warm with a dollop of Greek yogurt.

Note: Berry and Almond Crisp is a comforting and fruity dessert. The nutty almond topping adds crunch to the sweet and tart berries.

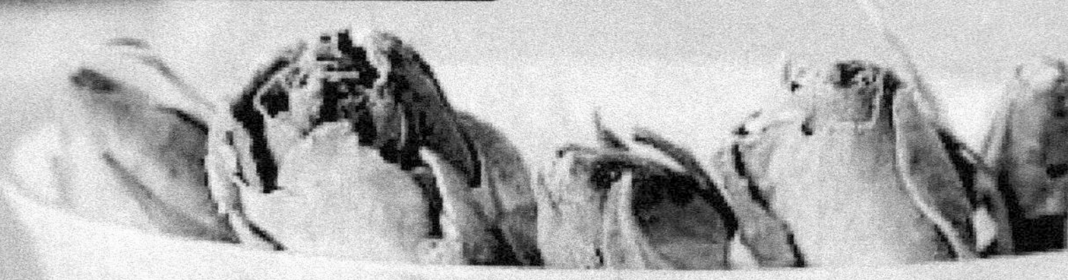

Chia Pudding Parfait: Healthy indulgence! 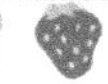

5.3 Chia Seed Pudding Parfait

SERVES: 2　　PREP TIME: 10 MIN　　CHILLING TIME: OVERNIGHT

INGREDIENTS

1/4 cup chia seeds
1 cup unsweetened almond milk
1 teaspoon vanilla extract
1 tablespoon maple syrup or sugar substitute
1 cup mixed berries (strawberries, blueberries, blackberries)
1/4 cup granola
Fresh mint for garnish

DIRECTIONS

1. In a jar, mix chia seeds, almond milk, vanilla extract, and maple syrup. Stir well and refrigerate overnight.
2. In serving glasses, layer chia pudding, mixed berries, and granola.
3. Garnish with fresh mint before serving.

Note:
Chia Seed Pudding Parfait is a delightful and nutrient-packed dessert. The layers of chia pudding, fresh berries, and granola create a parfait that's as visually appealing as it is delicious.

Sugar-Free Pumpkin Pie: Guilt-free treat!

5.4 Sugar-Free Pumpkin Pie

SERVES: 8   PREP TIME: 15 MIN   BAKING TIME: 45 MIN

INGREDIENTS

1 pre-made whole wheat pie crust

1 can pumpkin puree

1/2 cup unsweetened almond milk

2 large eggs

1 teaspoon pumpkin pie spice

1 teaspoon vanilla extract

1/4 cup sugar substitute

Whipped coconut cream for topping

DIRECTIONS

1. Preheat the oven to 350°F (180°C).
2. In a bowl, mix pumpkin puree, almond milk, eggs, pumpkin pie spice, vanilla extract, and sugar substitute until smooth.
3. Pour the mixture into the pie crust.
4. Bake for 40-45 minutes until the filling is set.
5. Allow the pie to cool before topping with whipped coconut cream.

Note:

Sugar-Free Pumpkin Pie offers all the flavors of the classic dessert without the added sugars. The creamy pumpkin filling in a whole wheat crust makes for a guilt-free and delicious treat.

Coconut Blueberry Muffins: Light & tasty!

5.5 Coconut Flour Blueberry Muffins

MAKES: 12 MUFFINS   PREP TIME: 15 MIN   BAKING TIME: 25 MIN

INGREDIENTS

1/2 cup coconut flour
1/2 teaspoon baking soda
Pinch of salt
4 large eggs
1/4 cup coconut oil, melted
1/4 cup unsweetened almond milk
1/4 cup maple syrup or sugar substitute
1 teaspoon vanilla extract
1 cup fresh blueberries

DIRECTIONS

1. Preheat the oven to 350°F (180°C) and line a muffin tin with paper liners.
2. In a bowl, whisk together coconut flour, baking soda, and salt.
3. In another bowl, beat eggs and add melted coconut oil, almond milk, maple syrup, and vanilla extract. Mix well.
4. Gradually add the dry ingredients to the wet ingredients and stir until combined.
5. Gently fold in the blueberries.
6. Spoon the batter into muffin cups and bake for 20-25 minutes until a toothpick comes out clean.

Note:
Sugar-Free Pumpkin Pie offers all the flavors of the classic dessert without the added sugars.

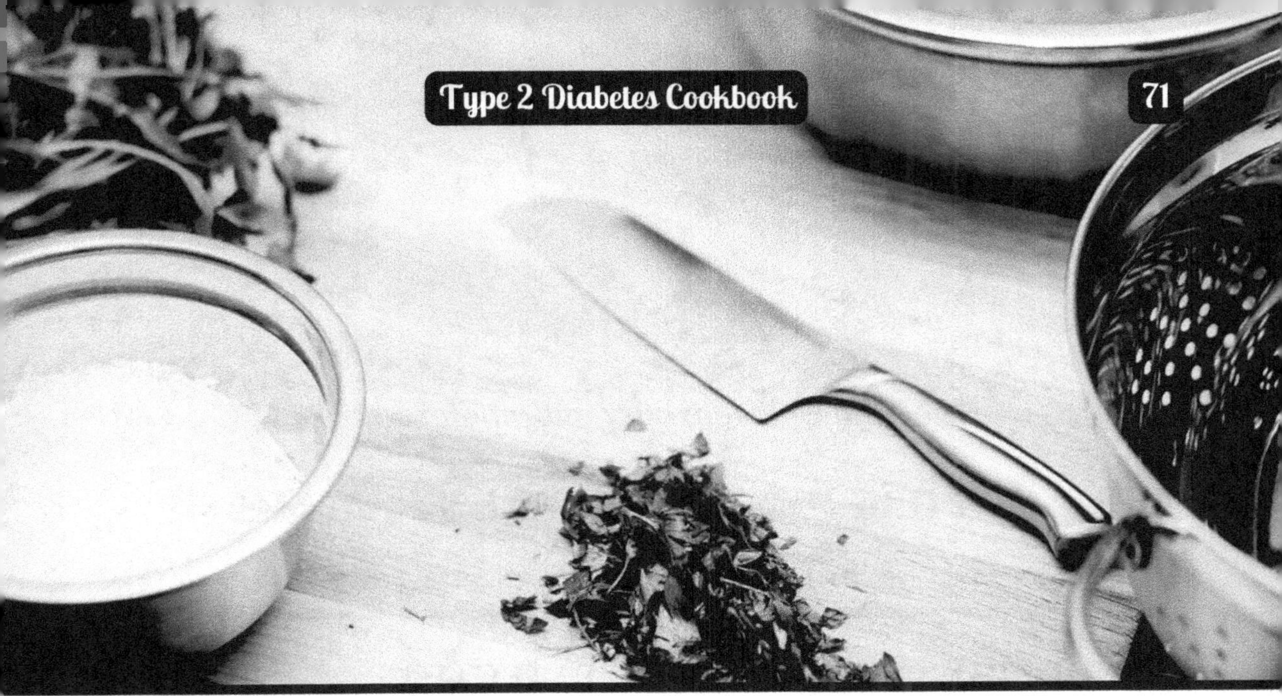

CHAPTER 6
ONE-POT WONDERS FOR DIABETES WELLNESS

Busy days necessitate quick and flavorful meals that don't skimp on nutrition. In this chapter, we'll look at one-pot marvels, which are simple, tasty foods that may be prepared in a single pot. From the simplicity of One-Pan Chicken and Vegetables to the heartiness of Lentil and Sweet Potato Stew, these dishes are intended to nourish your body while also saving you time in the kitchen.

Discover the simplicity of one-pot wonders with these diabetic-friendly recipes. From flavorful stews to fast stir-fries, these meals are designed to keep your diabetes under control while catering to your taste buds.

One-Pan Chicken: Easy and wholesome! 

6.1 One-Pan Chicken with Vegetables

SERVES: 4   **PREP TIME: 15 MIN**   **BAKING TIME: 30 MIN**

INGREDIENTS

4 boneless and skinless chicken breasts
1 pound baby potatoes (halved)
2 cups baby carrots.
1 cup trimmed green beans.
2 tablespoons olive oil
1 teaspoon garlic powder
1 teaspoon dried thyme
Add salt and pepper to taste
Garnish with fresh parsley

DIRECTIONS

1. Preheat your oven to 400°F (200°C).
2. In a mixing dish, combine chicken breasts, baby potatoes, baby carrots, and green beans with olive oil, garlic powder, dried thyme, salt, and pepper.
3. Spread the mixture onto a baking sheet and bake for 25-30 minutes, or until the chicken is fully cooked and the vegetables are soft.
4. Sprinkle with fresh parsley before serving.

Note:
One-Pan Chicken and Vegetables are a convenient and healthful meal alternative. The combination of lean protein and colorful vegetables makes it a well-balanced and diabetes-friendly meal.

Shrimp Quinoa Skillet: Quick and flavorful!

6.2 Shrimp & Quinoa Skillet

SERVES: 4   **PREP TIME: 10 MIN**   **COOK TIME: 20 MIN**

INGREDIENTS

1 cup rinsed quinoa
2 cups vegetable broth
1 pound peeled and deveined shrimp
1 cup halved cherry tomatoes
1 cup spinach
2 teaspoons olive oil.
2 garlic cloves, minced
1 teaspoon of smoked paprika
Add salt and pepper to taste
Serve with lemon wedges

DIRECTIONS

1. Cook the quinoa in a pan over medium heat until lightly brown.
2. Bring the vegetable stock to a boil, then reduce the heat and simmer for 15-20 minutes, or until the quinoa is cooked.
3. In a separate skillet, sauté shrimp, cherry tomatoes, and spinach in olive oil, minced garlic, smoked paprika, salt, and pepper until the shrimp are pink and the spinach has wilted.
4. Serve the shrimp and veggie mixture over cooked quinoa.
5. Squeeze lemon wedges over the meal before serving.

Note: Shrimp and Quinoa Skillet is a quick, protein-rich dinner. The combination of quinoa, shrimp, and vegetables results in a tasty and diabetes-friendly dinner.

Lentil Sweet Potato Stew: Hearty and nutritious!

6.3 Lentil & Sweet Potato Stew

SERVES: 6　　**PREP TIME: 15 MIN**　　**COOK TIME: 30 MIN**

INGREDIENTS

1 cup washed dry green lentils

2 diced sweet potatoes

1 chopped onion

3 minced garlic cloves.

1 can of diced tomatoes.

6 cups vegetable broth

1 teaspoon ground cumin

1 teaspoon smoky paprika.

Add salt and pepper to taste

Garnish with fresh cilantro.

DIRECTIONS

1. In a large pot, cook the onion and garlic until tender.
2. Combine the lentils, sweet potatoes, diced tomatoes, vegetable broth, cumin, smoky paprika, salt, and pepper. Bring to a boil.
3. Reduce the heat to a simmer for 25-30 minutes, or until the lentils and sweet potatoes are cooked.
4. Before serving, garnish with chopped fresh cilantro.

Note:

Lentil and Sweet Potato Stew is a hearty and satisfying one-pot meal. It's a soothing alternative for diabetics looking for a meal high in fiber and nutrients.

Mediterranean Chickpea Skillet: Flavorful & nutritious!

6.4 Mediterranean Chickpea Skillet

SERVES: 4　　　**PREP TIME: 10 MIN**　　　**COOK TIME: 15 MIN**

INGREDIENTS

2 tablespoons olive oil
1 chopped onion.
2 garlic cloves, minced
1 can (15 oz) drained chickpeas
1 can (14 oz) Diced tomatoes, unsweetened
1 cup quartered artichoke hearts and
1/2 cup sliced Kalamata olives
1 tsp dried oregano.
1 tsp dried basil
Season to taste with salt and pepper
Garnish with feta cheese and fresh parsley.

DIRECTIONS

1. Heat olive oil in a skillet and sauté the onion and garlic.
2. Add chickpeas, diced tomatoes, artichoke hearts, and olives, stirring to combine.
3. Season with oregano, basil, salt, and pepper, then simmer.
4. Just before serving, garnish with crumbled feta and fresh parsley.

Note:

Mediterranean Chickpea Skillet is a quick and savory choice that includes chickpeas, tomatoes, artichoke hearts, and olives. Crumbled feta serves as a finishing touch.

Easy Broccoli Cheese Casserole: Comfort in a dish!

6.5 Easy Broccoli & Cheese Casserole

SERVES: 6   **PREP TIME: 15 MIN**   **COOK TIME: 25 MIN**

INGREDIENTS

4 cups broccoli florets

1 cup shredded cheddar cheese

1/2 cup grated Parmesan cheese, and 1/2 cup Greek yogurt.

2 tablespoons whole wheat flour

2 tablespoons unsalted butter

1 cup unsweetened almond milk

2 garlic cloves, minced

Add salt and pepper to taste

Top with whole wheat breadcrumbs

DIRECTIONS

1. Heat the oven to 375°F (190°C) and butter a baking dish.
2. Steam the broccoli until just tender, then transfer it to the prepared baking dish.
3. Melt butter in a pot and cook minced garlic until fragrant.
4. Whisk in the whole wheat flour, then gradually add the almond milk, whisking constantly until thick.
5. Remove from heat and mix in the cheddar cheese, Parmesan cheese, Greek yogurt, salt, and pepper until smooth.
6. Drizzle the cheese mixture over the broccoli in the baking dish.
7. Sprinkle the top with whole wheat breadcrumbs.
8. Bake for 20-25 minutes, until the casserole is bubbling and brown.

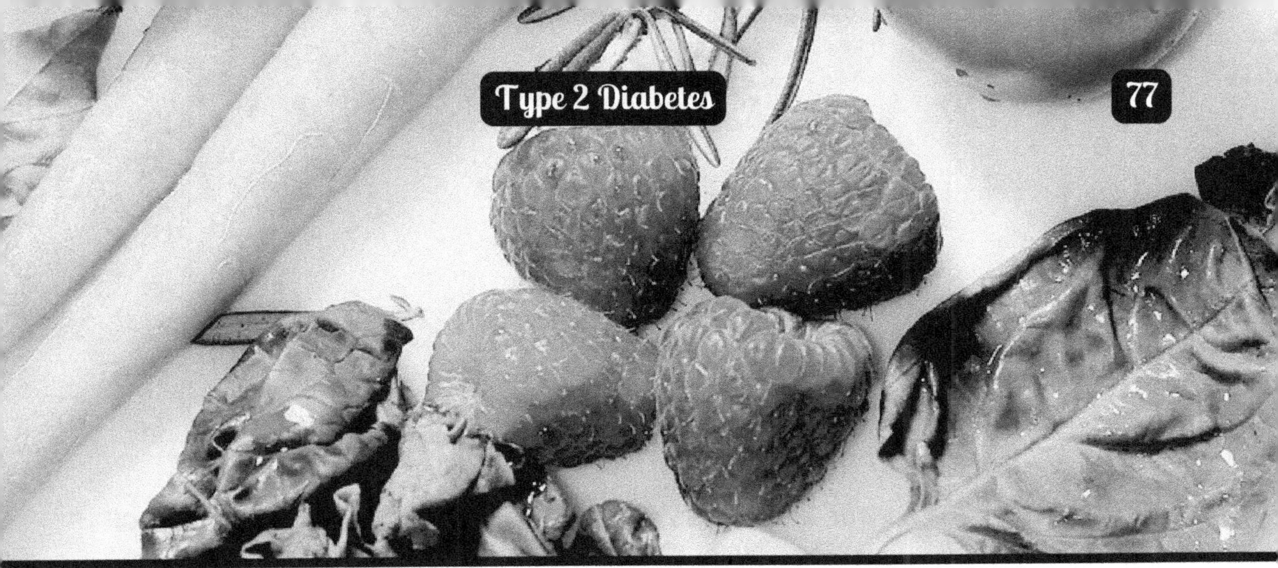

CHAPTER 7
VEGETARIAN & VEGAN OPTIONS FOR DIABETICS

Adopting a plant-based diet can be a beneficial option for managing diabetes. In this chapter, we'll look at a number of vegetarian and vegan meals that are both delicious and nutritious. These dishes, which range from the healthy Stuffed Bell Peppers to the savory Tofu and Vegetable Stir-Fry, are ideal for individuals looking for plant-based options for diabetes wellness.

Discover the world of vegetarian and vegan delights with these diabetic-friendly recipes. From protein-packed curries to vivid salads, these plant-powered options will nourish your body while also tantalizing your taste senses.

Quinoa Stuffed Peppers: Nutrient-packed goodness! 

7.1 Stuffed Bell Peppers with Quinoa & Black Beans

SERVES: 4   **PREP TIME: 20 MIN**   **COOK TIME: 35 MIN**

INGREDIENTS

4 halved bell peppers with seeds removed

1 cup cooked quinoa

1 can black beans (drained and rinsed)

1 cup corn kernels

1 cup diced tomatoes

1 teaspoon cumin

1 teaspoon chili powder.

Season to taste with salt and pepper.

Add 1 cup shredded vegan cheese (optional).

Fresh cilantro as garnish

DIRECTIONS

1. Preheat your oven to 375°F (190°C).
2. In a bowl, combine the cooked quinoa, black beans, corn, chopped tomatoes, cumin, chili powder, salt, and pepper.
3. Fill each bell pepper half with quinoa mixture.
4. Place the filled peppers on a baking tray, cover with foil, and bake for 25–30 minutes.
5. If using, sprinkle vegan cheese over the top and bake for an additional 5 minutes.
6. Before serving, garnish with chopped fresh cilantro.

Note:
Stuffed Bell Peppers with Quinoa and Black Beans provide a protein-rich and tasty dinner.

Lentil Spinach Curry: Spicy and wholesome!

7.2 Lentil & Spinach Curry

SERVES: 4   **PREP TIME: 15 MIN**   **COOK TIME: 30 MIN**

INGREDIENTS

1 cup rinsed dry green lentils

1 finely chopped onion

3 minced garlic cloves

1 tablespoon grated ginger

1 can diced tomatoes

2 cups spinach

1 can coconut milk.

1 tablespoon of curry powder.

1 teaspoon turmeric

Salt and pepper to taste

Garnish with fresh cilantro

DIRECTIONS

1. In a pot, cook the onion, garlic, and ginger until softened.
2. Combine the lentils, chopped tomatoes, spinach, coconut milk, curry powder, turmeric, salt, and pepper. Bring to a simmer.
3. Cover and simmer for 25-30 minutes, until lentils are cooked.
4. Before serving, garnish with chopped fresh cilantro.

Note:

Lentil and Spinach Curry is a filling and fragrant dish. It's a satisfying alternative for people wishing to add more vegetarian meals into their diabetes-friendly diet, thanks to its high plant-based protein content.

Roasted Veg Chickpea Salad: Fresh & flavorful! 🥗🥒

7.3 Roasted Veggie & Chickpea Salad

SERVES: 4　　　　**PREP TIME: 15 MIN**　　　　**COOK TIME: 25 MIN**

INGREDIENTS

2 cups of mixed veggies (zucchini, cherry tomatoes, bell peppers) chopped
1 can of chickpeas drained and rinsed
2 tablespoons olive oil
1 teaspoon dried oregano.
1 teaspoon of smoked paprika.
Season with salt and pepper to taste
Serve with mixed salad greens and balsamic vinaigrette dressing

DIRECTIONS

1. Preheat your oven to 400°F (200°C).
2. In a mixing dish, combine the veggies and chickpeas with olive oil, dried oregano, smoked paprika, salt, and pepper.
3. Place the mixture on a baking sheet and roast for 20-25 minutes, until the veggies are soft.
4. Spread the roasted veggies and chickpeas on a bed of mixed salad greens.
5. Drizzle with balsamic vinaigrette before serving.

Note:
Roasted vegetable and chickpea salad is a colorful and nutrient-dense choice. The mix of roasted vegetables and protein-rich chickpeas yields a filling salad for diabetic management.

Tofu Veg Stir-Fry: Tasty plant-powered delight!

7.4 Tofu & Vegetable Stir-fry

SERVES: 4　　　**PREP TIME: 15 MIN**　　　**COOK TIME: 15 MIN**

INGREDIENTS

1 block firm tofu, cubed
2 cups broccoli florets
1 sliced bell pepper
1 cup snap peas
2 tsp low-sodium soy sauce
1 tbsp hoisin sauce
1 tbsp sesame oil
1 tbsp rice vinegar
1 tbsp maple syrup or sugar replacement
2 garlic cloves, minced
1 tsp grated ginger
Garnish with sesame seeds and green onions.

DIRECTIONS

1. Brown tofu in a wok or skillet, then set aside.
2. Sauté broccoli, bell pepper, and snap peas until crisp-tender.
3. Mix soy sauce, hoisin sauce, sesame oil, rice vinegar, maple syrup, garlic, and ginger in a bowl.
4. Add tofu back to the pan, pour in the sauce, and stir well.
5. Garnish with sesame seeds and green onions before serving.

Note:
Tofu and Vegetable Stir-Fry is a simple and flavorful plant-based protein dish. The variety of bright vegetables makes it both visually appealing and diabetic-friendly.

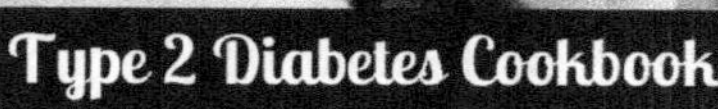

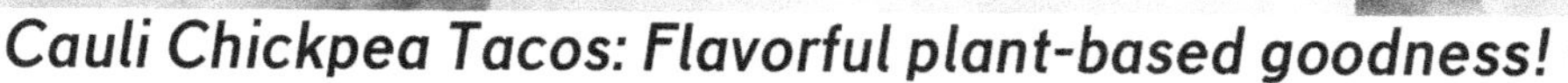

Cauli Chickpea Tacos: Flavorful plant-based goodness!

7.5 Cauliflower & Chickpea Tacos

SERVES: 4   PREP TIME: 15 MIN   COOK TIME: 30 MIN

INGREDIENTS

1 head cauliflower, chopped into florets
1 can chickpeas, drained and rinsed 2 tablespoons olive oil
1 teaspoon cumin
1 teaspoon chili powder
1/2 teaspoon of smoked paprika
Season with salt and pepper to taste
Top with avocado slices and garnish with fresh cilantro
Serve over corn tortillas

DIRECTIONS

1. Pre-heat the oven to 425°F (220°C).
2. In a mixing dish, combine cauliflower florets and chickpeas with olive oil, cumin, chili powder, smoked paprika, salt, and pepper.
3. Place the mixture on a baking sheet and roast for 25-30 minutes, until the cauliflower is golden and the chickpeas are crispy.
4. Add avocado slices and garnish with fresh cilantro
5. Serve the roasted cauliflower and chickpeas in corn tortillas

Note:

Cauliflower and Chickpea Tacos are a great, meatless option. For diabetic taco lovers, the roasted cauliflower and spicy chickpeas make a delightful filler.

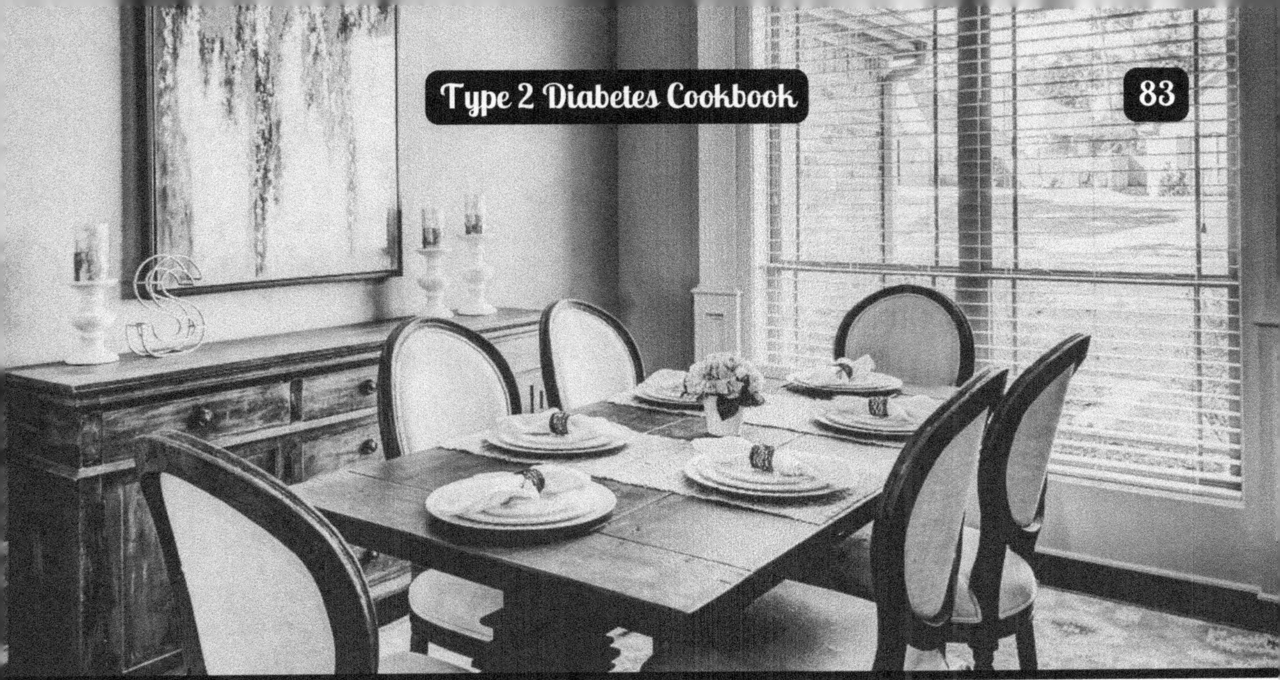

CHAPTER 8
FAMILY-FRIENDLY DIABETIC DINNERS

It is not difficult to prepare meals that are suitable for the entire family while keeping to diabetes treatment guidelines. This chapter contains a variety of family-friendly dinner recipes that are both delicious and low in blood sugar. From the delectable Turkey and Vegetable Meatballs to the engaging Balanced Taco Night, these recipes strive to make dinnertime fun and healthy for everyone.

Make family dinners a happy experience with these diabetes-friendly dishes.

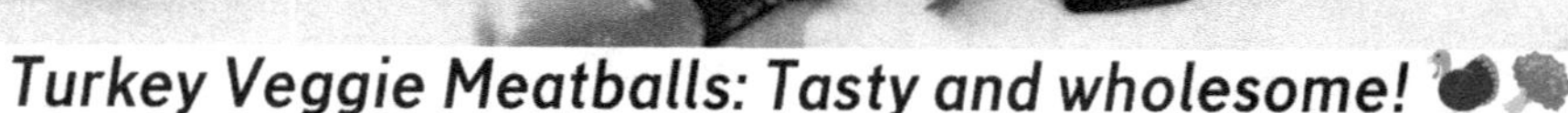

Turkey Veggie Meatballs: Tasty and wholesome!

8.1 Turkey & Vegetable Meatballs

SERVES: 4   PREP TIME: 15 MIN   BAKING TIME: 25 MIN

INGREDIENTS

1 pound lean ground turkey
1/2 cup grated zucchini
1/2 cup grated carrot
1/4 cup whole wheat breadcrumbs
1/4 cup grated Parmesan cheese
1 egg
2 cloves garlic, minced
1 teaspoon dried oregano
1 teaspoon dried basil
Salt and pepper to taste
Marinara sauce for serving

DIRECTIONS

1. Preheat the oven to 375°F (190°C).
2. In a bowl, mix ground turkey, grated zucchini, grated carrot, breadcrumbs, Parmesan cheese, egg, minced garlic, oregano, basil, salt, and pepper.
3. Shape the mixture into meatballs and place on a baking sheet.
4. Bake for 20-25 minutes until meatballs are cooked through.
5. Serve with marinara sauce.

Note:
Turkey and Vegetable Meatballs offer a lean and flavorful alternative to traditional meatballs. The addition of veggies enhances the nutritional value, making it a hit for family dinners.

Mini Whole Wheat Pita Pizzas: Bite-sized pizza bliss!

8.2 Mini Pita Pizzas with Whole Wheat Crust

SERVES: 6   **PREP TIME: 10 MIN**   **BAKING TIME: 12 MIN**

INGREDIENTS

Whole wheat mini pitas
1 cup tomato sauce (low-sugar or homemade)
1 cup part-skim mozzarella cheese, shredded
Assorted vegetable toppings (bell peppers, cherry tomatoes, mushrooms)
Turkey pepperoni slices (optional)
Fresh basil for garnish

DIRECTIONS

1. Preheat the oven to 375°F (190°C).
2. Place whole wheat mini pitas on a baking sheet.
3. Spread a thin layer of tomato sauce on each pita.
4. Sprinkle shredded mozzarella cheese over the sauce.
5. Add assorted vegetable toppings and turkey pepperoni slices if desired.
6. Bake for 10-12 minutes until the cheese is melted and bubbly.
7. Garnish with fresh basil before serving.

Note:
Mini Pita Pizzas with Whole Wheat Crust provide a fun and customizable dinner option for the whole family. Let everyone choose their favorite toppings for a personalized touch.

Baked Chicken Tenders: Sweet Potato Fries. 

8.3 Baked Chicken Tenders with Sweet Potato Fries

SERVES: 4   PREP TIME: 15 MIN   BAKING TIME: 25 MIN

INGREDIENTS

Chicken tenders
1 cup whole wheat
breadcrumbs
1/4 cup grated
Parmesan cheese
1 teaspoon garlic
powder
1 teaspoon paprika
Salt and pepper to
taste
Sweet potatoes, cut
into fries
2 tablespoons olive
oil
1/2 teaspoon smoked
paprika
1/2 teaspoon cumin
Greek yogurt
dipping sauce

DIRECTIONS

1. Preheat the oven to 400°F (200°C).
2. In a bowl, mix whole wheat breadcrumbs, grated Parmesan cheese, garlic powder, paprika, salt, and pepper.
3. Dip chicken tenders into the breadcrumb mixture, ensuring they are coated evenly, and place on a baking sheet.
4. In a separate bowl, toss sweet potato fries with olive oil, smoked paprika, and cumin. Spread on the baking sheet.
5. Bake for 20-25 minutes until chicken is cooked through and sweet potato fries are crispy.
6. Serve with a side of Greek yogurt dipping sauce.

Veggie Spaghetti Sauce: Packed with goodness!

8.4 Veggie-Packed Spaghetti Sauce

SERVES: 4 **PREP TIME: 15 MIN** **COOK TIME: 20 MIN**

INGREDIENTS

1 pound whole wheat spaghetti
1 tablespoon olive oil
1 onion, finely chopped
2 carrots, grated
2 zucchinis, grated
3 cloves garlic, minced
1 can crushed tomatoes
1 can tomato paste
1 teaspoon dried oregano
1 teaspoon dried basil
Salt and pepper to taste
Fresh parsley for garnish

DIRECTIONS

1. Cook whole wheat spaghetti according to package instructions.
2. In a large saucepan, heat olive oil and sauté chopped onion, grated carrots, grated zucchinis, and minced garlic until softened.
3. Add crushed tomatoes, tomato paste, dried oregano, dried basil, salt, and pepper. Simmer for 15-20 minutes.
4. Serve the veggie-packed sauce over cooked whole wheat spaghetti.
5. Garnish with fresh parsley before serving.

Note:
Veggie-Packed Spaghetti Sauce is a nutritious and flavorful twist on a classic family dinner. Sneak in extra veggies without compromising on taste.

Balanced Taco Night: Flavorful and wholesome!

8.5 Balanced Taco Night

SERVES: 4   **PREP TIME: 15 MIN**   **COOK TIME: 10 MIN**

INGREDIENTS

Lean ground turkey or chicken

Whole wheat taco shells or lettuce wraps

Black beans, drained and rinsed

Diced tomatoes

Shredded lettuce

Shredded cheddar cheese

Greek yogurt or low-fat sour cream

Salsa

Avocado slices

Fresh cilantro for garnish

DIRECTIONS

1. In a skillet, cook lean ground turkey or chicken until browned.
2. Warm whole wheat taco shells or prepare lettuce wraps.
3. Set up a taco station with black beans, diced tomatoes, shredded lettuce, shredded cheddar cheese, Greek yogurt or low-fat sour cream, salsa, avocado slices, and fresh cilantro.
4. Let each family member build their own balanced tacos.

Note:

Balanced Taco Night is an interactive and customizable dinner option for the entire family. It allows everyone to tailor their tacos to their liking while keeping it diabetes-friendly.

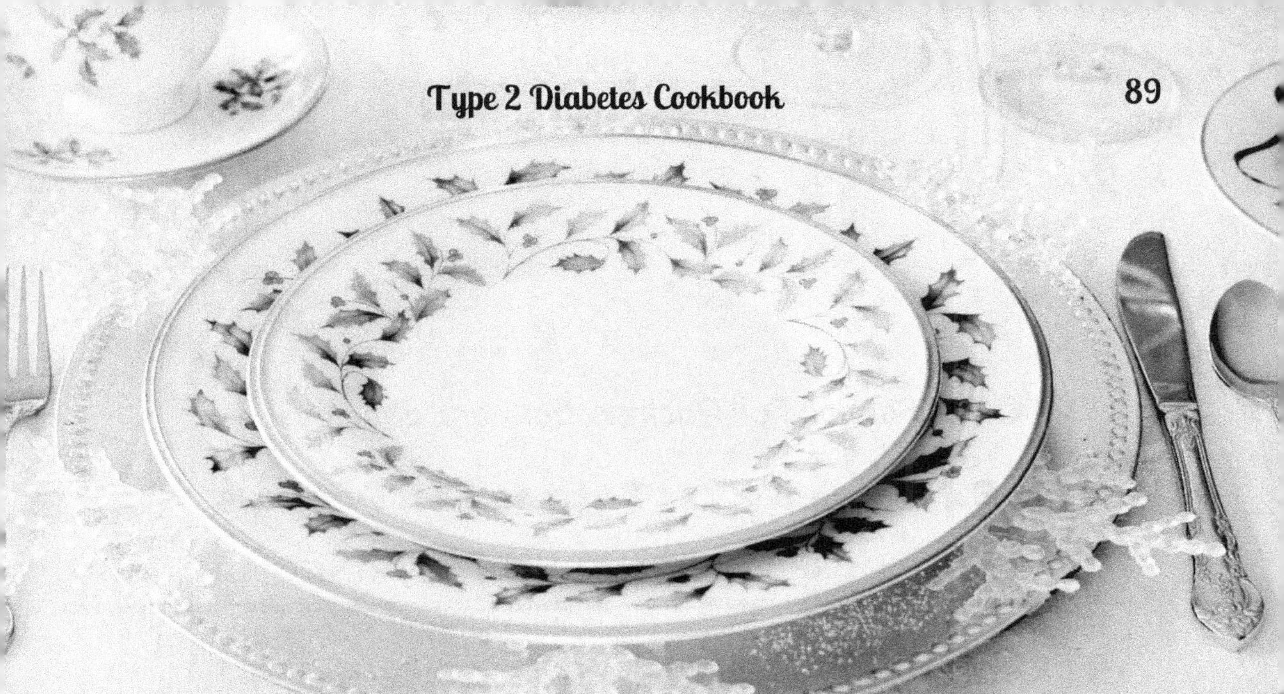

CHAPTER 9
30-MINUTE DIABETIC DINNERS

For those hectic evenings when time is of the utmost, this chapter contains a range of quick and delicious dinners that may be on the table in under 30 minutes. From the fuss-free Quick and Easy Salmon Foil Packets to the zesty Rapid Veggie and Sausage Sheet Pan Dinner, these dishes ensure that diabetes management does not take up your valuable time.

Explore the convenience of these 30-minute diabetic dinners, which ensure that health-conscious options need not sacrifice taste or satisfaction. Whether it's the simplicity of salmon foil packets or the quickness of chicken tacos, these recipes make diabetes management a breeze on hectic evenings.

Quick Salmon Foil Packets: Easy and delicious!

9.1 Quick & Easy Salmon Foil Packets

SERVES: 4   **PREP TIME: 10 MIN**   **BAKING TIME: 20 MIN**

INGREDIENTS

4 salmon fillets
2 cups mixed vegetables (zucchini, cherry tomatoes, bell peppers)
2 tablespoons olive oil
1 lemon, sliced
2 cloves garlic, minced
1 teaspoon dried dill
Salt and pepper to taste

DIRECTIONS

1. Preheat the oven to 400°F (200°C).
2. Place each salmon fillet on a piece of foil.
3. Divide mixed vegetables among the foil packets, arranging them around the salmon.
4. Drizzle olive oil over the salmon and vegetables.
5. Sprinkle minced garlic, dried dill, salt, and pepper.
6. Place lemon slices on top of each salmon fillet.
7. Seal the foil packets and bake for 20 minutes until salmon is cooked through and vegetables are tender.

Note: Quick and Easy Salmon Foil Packets simplify dinner preparation without sacrificing flavor.

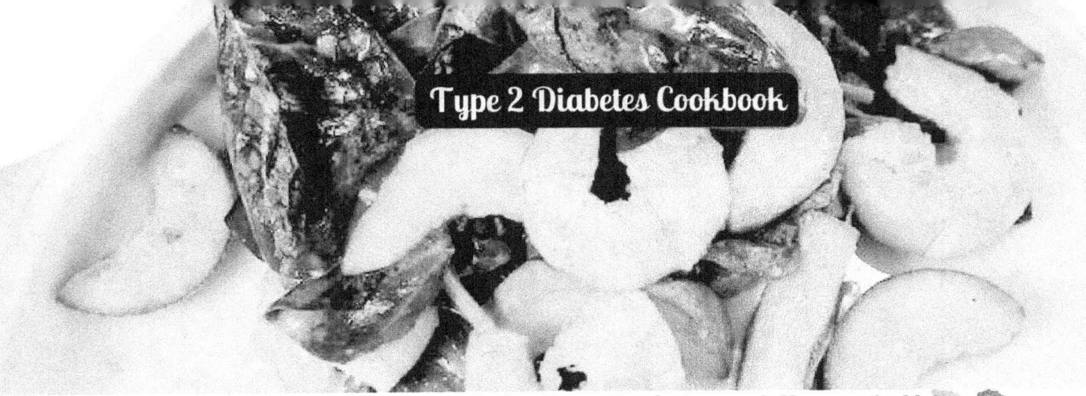

Speedy Shrimp Stir-Fry: Quick and flavorful!

9.2 Speedy Vegetable Stir-Fry with Shrimp

SERVES: 4   PREP TIME: 15 MIN   COOKING TIME: 15 MIN

INGREDIENTS

1 lb shrimp, peeled and deveined
4 cups mixed vegetables (broccoli, bell peppers, snap peas)
2 tbsp low-sodium soy sauce
1 tbsp sesame oil
1 tbsp rice vinegar
1 tbsp honey or sugar substitute
2 cloves garlic, minced
1 tsp grated ginger
2 green onions, sliced
Sesame seeds for garnish
Cooked brown rice for serving

DIRECTIONS

1. Stir-fry shrimp until pink; set aside.
2. Stir-fry mixed vegetables until crisp-tender.
3. Whisk soy sauce, sesame oil, rice vinegar, honey, garlic, and ginger in a bowl.
4. Add cooked shrimp back, pour sauce, stir to coat.
5. Garnish with green onions and sesame seeds.
6. Serve over brown rice.

Note:

Speedy Vegetable Stir-Fry with Shrimp is a quick and flavorful option for a diabetes-friendly dinner. The colorful veggies and protein-packed shrimp create a balanced and satisfying meal.

Simple Turkey Quinoa Skillet: Easy and nutritious! 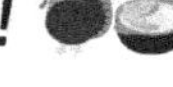

9.3 Simple Turkey & Quinoa Skillet

SERVES: 4   PREP TIME: 10 MIN   COOKING TIME: 15 MIN

INGREDIENTS

1 pound lean ground turkey

1 cup quinoa, cooked

2 cups mixed vegetables (peas, carrots, corn)

1 can diced tomatoes

1 teaspoon dried oregano

1 teaspoon ground cumin

Salt and pepper to taste

Fresh parsley for garnish

DIRECTIONS

1. In a large skillet, cook lean ground turkey until browned.
2. Add cooked quinoa, mixed vegetables, diced tomatoes, dried oregano, ground cumin, salt, and pepper. Stir to combine.
3. Simmer for 10-15 minutes until the flavors meld and the mixture is heated through.
4. Garnish with fresh parsley before serving.

Note:

Simple Turkey and Quinoa Skillet offer a wholesome and speedy option for a diabetes-friendly dinner. The combination of lean turkey and quinoa provides a protein-packed and satisfying meal.

Quick Beef Stir-Fry: Speedy and savory!

9.4 Quick Beef Stir-Fry

SERVES: 4   **PREP TIME: 15 MIN**   **COOKING TIME: 15 MIN**

INGREDIENTS

1 lb lean beef strips
2 cups broccoli florets
1 sliced carrot, 1 sliced bell pepper
2 tbsp low-sodium soy sauce
1 tbsp each oyster sauce, sesame oil, rice vinegar
1 tbsp honey or sugar substitute
2 cloves garlic, minced; 1 tsp grated ginger
2 sliced green onions; Sesame seeds
Cooked brown rice for serving

DIRECTIONS

1. Stir-fry beef until browned; set aside.
2. Stir-fry broccoli, carrot, and bell pepper until crisp-tender.
3. Whisk soy sauce, oyster sauce, sesame oil, rice vinegar, honey, garlic, and ginger in a bowl.
4. Add cooked beef back, pour sauce, stir.
5. Garnish with green onions and sesame seeds.
6. Serve over brown rice.

Note:

Quick and savory, this Easy Beef Stir-Fry is a delightful and nutritious option for a diabetes-friendly dinner.

Rapid Veggie Sausage Dinner: Sheet pan perfection!

9.5 Rapid Veggie & Sausage Sheet Pan Dinner

SERVES: 4　　　**PREP TIME: 10 MIN**　　　**ROASTING TIME: 25 MIN**

INGREDIENTS

4 chicken sausages, sliced

4 cups mixed vegetables (potatoes, bell peppers, broccoli)

2 tablespoons olive oil

1 teaspoon dried thyme

1 teaspoon dried rosemary

Salt and pepper to taste

Balsamic glaze for drizzling

DIRECTIONS

1. Preheat the oven to 425°F (220°C).
2. On a sheet pan, arrange sliced chicken sausages and mixed vegetables.
3. Drizzle with olive oil and sprinkle dried thyme, dried rosemary, salt, and pepper. Toss to coat evenly.
4. Roast in the oven for 20-25 minutes until sausages are cooked through and vegetables are golden.
5. Drizzle with balsamic glaze before serving.

Note:

Rapid Veggie and Sausage Sheet Pan Dinner is a convenient and flavorful choice for a diabetes-friendly dinner. The balsamic glaze adds a touch of sweetness to this quick and nutritious sheet pan meal.

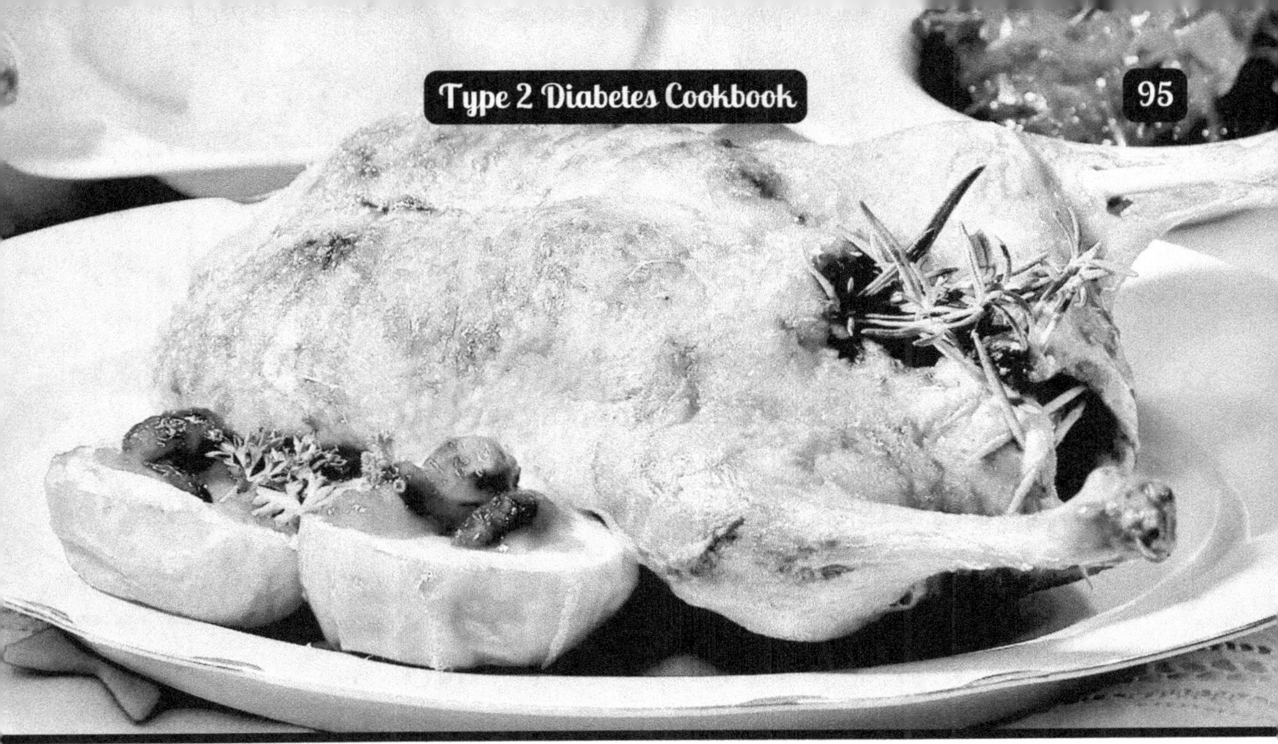

CHAPTER 10
HOLIDAY FEASTS FOR DIABETICS

Meant for the holiday season, this chapter is dedicated to creating festive feasts that celebrate the joy of gatherings without compromising on diabetes-conscious choices. From the centerpiece Herb-Roasted Turkey with Cranberry Relish to the delectable Sugar-Free Pumpkin Cheesecake, these recipes ensure that the holiday table is filled with flavor and health.

Elevate your holiday celebrations with these festive feasts that cater to diabetes-conscious choices without compromising on the joy and flavor of the season. Each recipe is crafted to make your holiday gatherings memorable and health-conscious.

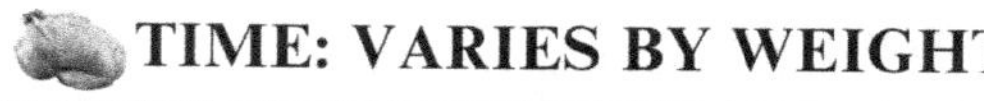

Herb-Roasted Turkey: Cranberry perfection!

10.1 Herb-Roasted Turkey with Cranberry Relish

SERVES: 12-15 PREP TIME: 20 MIN   TIME: VARIES BY WEIGHT

INGREDIENTS

1 whole turkey (12-15 pounds)
1/4 cup olive oil
2 tablespoons fresh rosemary, chopped
2 tablespoons fresh thyme, chopped
Salt and pepper to taste
Cranberry relish for serving

DIRECTIONS

1. Preheat the oven to 325°F (163°C).
2. In a small bowl, mix olive oil, chopped rosemary, chopped thyme, salt, and pepper.
3. Place the turkey on a rack in a roasting pan.
4. Rub the herb mixture over the turkey, ensuring an even coating.
5. Roast the turkey in the preheated oven, following recommended cooking times based on weight.
6. Allow the turkey to rest before carving.
7. Serve with cranberry relish.

Note: Turkey with Cranberry Relish provides a centerpiece for your holiday feast that is both succulent and diabetes-friendly.

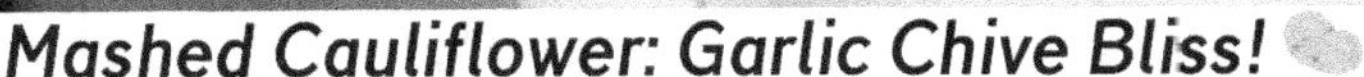

Mashed Cauliflower: Garlic Chive Bliss!

10.2 Mashed Cauliflower with Garlic & Chives

SERVES: 6　　　**PREP TIME: 15 MIN**　　　**ROASTING TIME: 15 MIN**

INGREDIENTS

1 large head cauliflower, cut into florets
2 cloves garlic, minced
2 tablespoons unsalted butter
1/4 cup Greek yogurt
Salt and pepper to taste
Fresh chives for garnish

DIRECTIONS

1. Steam or boil cauliflower florets until tender.
2. In a food processor, blend cauliflower, minced garlic, butter, Greek yogurt, salt, and pepper until smooth.
3. Adjust seasoning to taste.
4. Garnish with fresh chives before serving.

Note:
Mashed Cauliflower with Garlic and Chives offers a low-carb and flavorful alternative to traditional mashed potatoes, making it a perfect side dish for your holiday feast.

Green Beans Almondine: Nutty goodness! 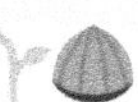

10.3 Green Beans Almondine

SERVES: 4   PREP TIME: 10 MIN   COOKING TIME: 10 MIN

INGREDIENTS

1 pound fresh green beans, trimmed
2 tablespoons olive oil
1/4 cup sliced almonds
2 cloves garlic, minced
Salt and pepper to taste
Lemon zest for garnish

DIRECTIONS

1. Blanch green beans in boiling water for 2-3 minutes until crisp-tender. Drain and set aside.
2. In a skillet, heat olive oil over medium heat.
3. Add sliced almonds and sauté until golden.
4. Add minced garlic and sauté for 1 minute.
5. Add blanched green beans, tossing to coat in the almond-garlic mixture.
6. Season with salt and pepper.
7. Transfer to a serving dish and garnish with lemon zest.

Note:

Green Beans Almondine provides a vibrant and nutty side dish that adds a burst of color and flavor to your holiday table while keeping it diabetes-friendly.

Sugar-Free Pumpkin Cheesecake: Guilt-free delight! 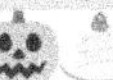

10.4 Sugar-Free Pumpkin Cheesecake

SERVES: 12   PREP TIME: 20 MIN   BAKING TIME: 50-60 MIN

INGREDIENTS

2 cups almond flour
1/2 cup unsalted butter, melted
4 packages (32 ounces) cream cheese, softened
1 cup pumpkin puree
1 cup granulated sugar substitute
4 large eggs
1 teaspoon vanilla extract
1 teaspoon pumpkin spice
Whipped cream for garnish

DIRECTIONS

1. Preheat the oven to 325°F (163°C).
2. In a bowl, combine almond flour and melted butter to create the crust. Press into the bottom of a springform pan.
3. In a large mixing bowl, beat cream cheese until smooth.
4. Add pumpkin puree, sugar substitute, eggs, vanilla extract, and pumpkin spice. Mix until well combined.
5. Pour the cream cheese mixture over the crust.
6. Bake in the preheated oven for 50-60 minutes or until the center is set.
7. Allow the cheesecake to cool before refrigerating for at least 4 hours or overnight.
8. Serve chilled, garnished with whipped cream.

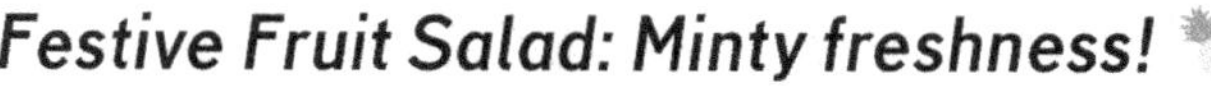

Festive Fruit Salad: Minty freshness!

10.5 Festive Fruit Salad with Mint

SERVES: 6   **PREP TIME: 10 MIN**   **COOKING TIME: 0 MIN**

INGREDIENTS

4 cups mixed fresh fruit (berries, citrus segments, kiwi)
2 tablespoons fresh orange juice
1 tablespoon honey or sugar substitute
Fresh mint leaves for garnish

DIRECTIONS

1. In a large bowl, combine mixed fresh fruit.
2. In a small bowl, whisk together fresh orange juice and honey or sugar substitute.
3. Drizzle the orange juice mixture over the fruit and toss gently to coat.
4. Garnish with fresh mint leaves before serving.

Note:
Festive Fruit Salad with Mint brings a refreshing and colorful touch to your holiday table. The citrusy dressing enhances the natural sweetness of the fruit while maintaining a diabetes-conscious choice.

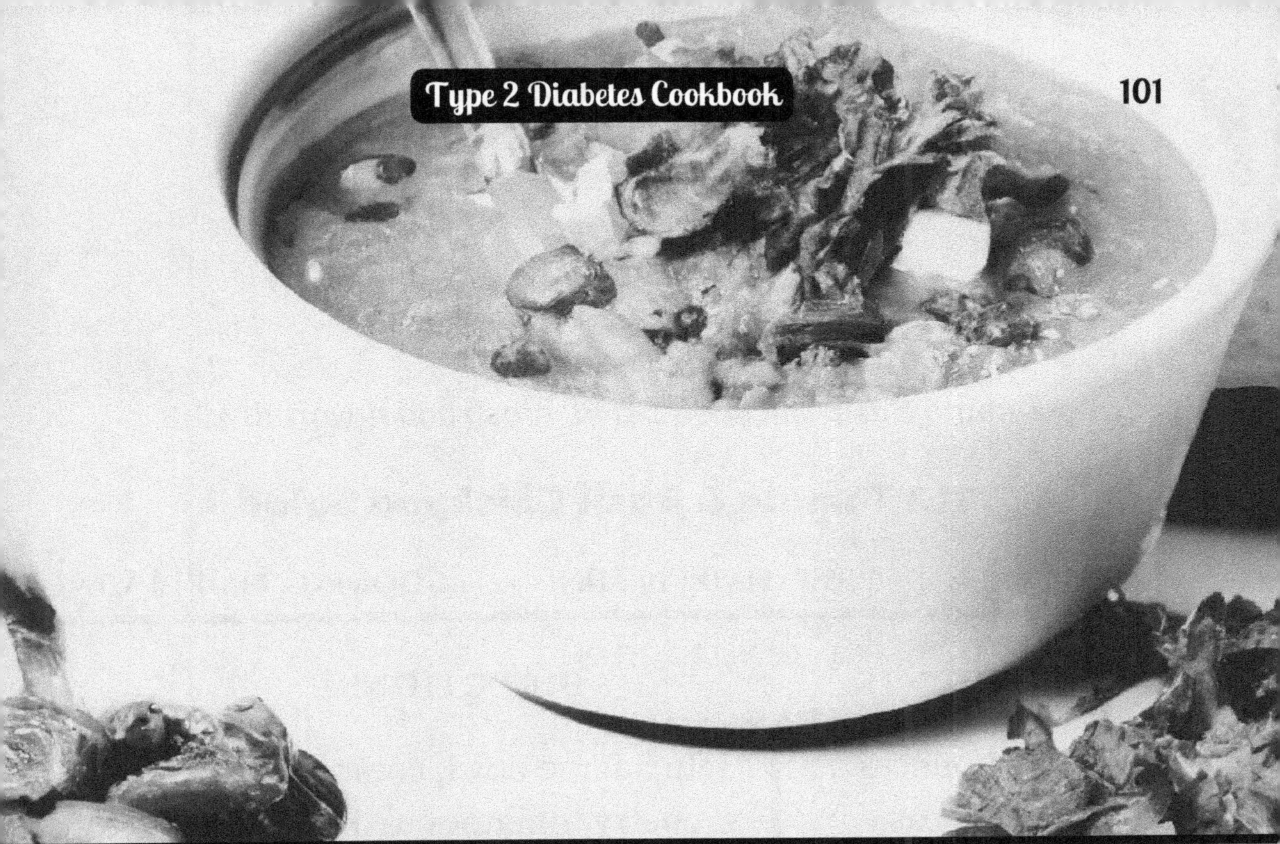

CHAPTER 11
BUDGET-FRIENDLY DIABETIC RECIPES

Healthy eating does not have to be expensive. In this chapter, we'll look at diabetic meals that are both economical and delicious. From the nourishing Lentil and Vegetable Soup to the soothing Broccoli and Cheddar Stuffed Baked Potatoes, these dishes demonstrate that diabetes management can be both cost-effective and gratifying.

Tomato Basil Chickpea Salad: Fresh and flavorful! 🍅🌿

11.1 Tomato & Basil Chickpea Salad

SERVES: 4   **PREP TIME: 10 MIN**   **COOKING TIME: 0 MIN**

INGREDIENTS

2 cans (15 ounces each) chickpeas, drained and rinsed

2 cups cherry tomatoes, halved

1/2 cup red onion, finely chopped

1/4 cup fresh basil, chopped

2 tablespoons olive oil

1 tablespoon balsamic vinegar

Salt and pepper to taste

Feta cheese crumbles for garnish

DIRECTIONS

1. In a large bowl, combine chickpeas, cherry tomatoes, red onion, and fresh basil.
2. In a small bowl, whisk together olive oil, balsamic vinegar, salt, and pepper.
3. Pour the dressing over the chickpea mixture and toss to coat.
4. Garnish with feta cheese crumbles before serving.

Note:

Tomato and Basil Chickpea Salad presents a refreshing and budget-friendly option for a diabetes-conscious side dish or light meal. The combination of chickpeas, tomatoes, and basil creates a simple yet flavorful salad.

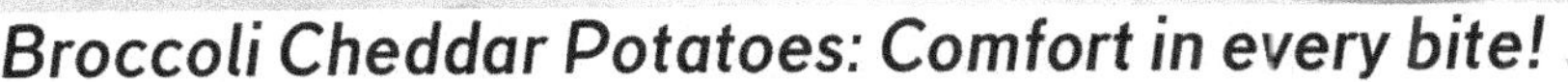

Broccoli Cheddar Potatoes: Comfort in every bite!

11.2 Broccoli & Cheddar Stuffed Baked Potatoes

SERVES: 4   **PREP TIME: 15 MIN**   **BAKING TIME: 0 MIN**

INGREDIENTS

4 medium-sized russet potatoes, scrubbed
2 cups broccoli florets, steamed
1 cup shredded sharp cheddar cheese
1/2 cup plain Greek yogurt
2 green onions, sliced
Salt and pepper to taste

DIRECTIONS

1. Preheat the oven to 400°F (200°C).
2. Pierce each potato several times with a fork and bake for 45-60 minutes until tender.
3. Cut a slit in each baked potato and fluff the insides with a fork.
4. In a bowl, mix steamed broccoli, shredded cheddar cheese, Greek yogurt, sliced green onions, salt, and pepper.
5. Spoon the broccoli and cheddar mixture into each baked potato.
6. Return to the oven for 10 minutes until the cheese is melted.
7. Serve warm.

Note: Broccoli and Cheddar Stuffed Baked Potatoes offer a comforting and budget-friendly option for a diabetes-friendly meal.

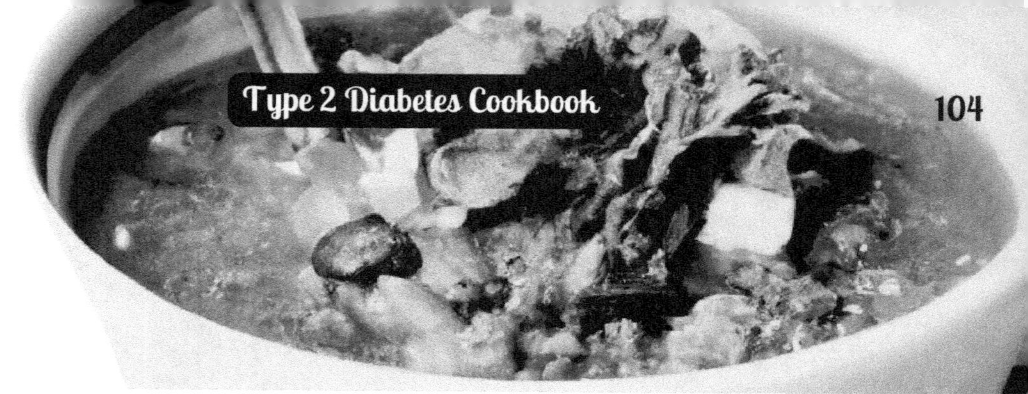

Budget Turkey Chili: Affordable and delicious! 

11.3 Budget-Friendly Turkey Chili

SERVES: 6   **PREP TIME: 15 MIN**   **COOKING TIME: 25 MIN**

INGREDIENTS

1 lb lean ground turkey
1 onion, chopped
2 bell peppers, diced
3 cloves garlic, minced
1 can (14 oz) kidney beans, black beans, diced tomatoes
2 cups low-sodium tomato juice
2 tbsp chili powder
1 tsp cumin, smoked paprika
- Salt and pepper to taste
- Fresh cilantro for garnish

DIRECTIONS

1. Brown turkey in a pot.
2. Add onion, bell peppers, and garlic; cook until softened.
3. Stir in beans, tomatoes, tomato juice, spices; simmer 20-25 minutes.
4. Adjust seasoning.
5. Garnish with fresh cilantro before serving.

Note:

Budget-Friendly Turkey Chili is a hearty and economical choice for a diabetes-conscious meal. Packed with protein and fiber, this chili satisfies both the palate and the budget.

Easy Cabbage Sausage Skillet: Quick and tasty! 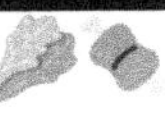

11.4 Easy Cabbage & Sausage Skillet

SERVES: 4　　　　**PREP TIME: 10 MIN**　　　　**COOKING TIME: 20 MIN**

INGREDIENTS

1 pound turkey or chicken sausage, sliced

1 head cabbage, thinly sliced

1 onion, thinly sliced

2 cloves garlic, minced

1 teaspoon caraway seeds

Salt and pepper to taste

Fresh parsley for garnish

DIRECTIONS

1. In a large skillet, brown sliced sausage over medium heat.
2. Add thinly sliced cabbage, sliced onion, minced garlic, caraway seeds, salt, and pepper.
3. Cook, stirring occasionally, until the cabbage is tender and slightly caramelized.
4. Adjust seasoning to taste.
5. Garnish with fresh parsley before serving.

Note:

Easy Cabbage and Sausage Skillet offers a simple yet flavorful option for a budget-friendly diabetes-conscious meal. The combination of cabbage and sausage creates a satisfying and nutritious skillet dish.

Economical Egg Casserole: Affordable and nutritious! 🔍

11.5 Economical Egg & Vegetable Casserole

SERVES: 6　　　**PREP TIME: 15 MIN**　　　**BAKING TIME: 30-35 MIN**

INGREDIENTS

8 eggs
1 cup milk (dairy or non-dairy)
1 cup diced bell peppers
1 cup diced zucchini
1 cup cherry tomatoes, halved
1 cup shredded sharp cheddar cheese
1 teaspoon dried oregano
Salt and pepper to taste
Fresh chives for garnish

DIRECTIONS

1. Preheat the oven to 375°F (190°C). Grease a baking dish.
2. In a bowl, whisk together eggs, milk, diced bell peppers, diced zucchini, cherry tomatoes, shredded cheddar cheese, dried oregano, salt, and pepper.
3. Pour the mixture into the prepared baking dish.
4. Bake for 30-35 minutes or until the casserole is set and lightly golden.
5. Garnish with fresh chives before serving.

Note:

Economical Egg and Vegetable Casserole provides a protein-packed and budget-friendly option for a diabetes-conscious breakfast or brunch.

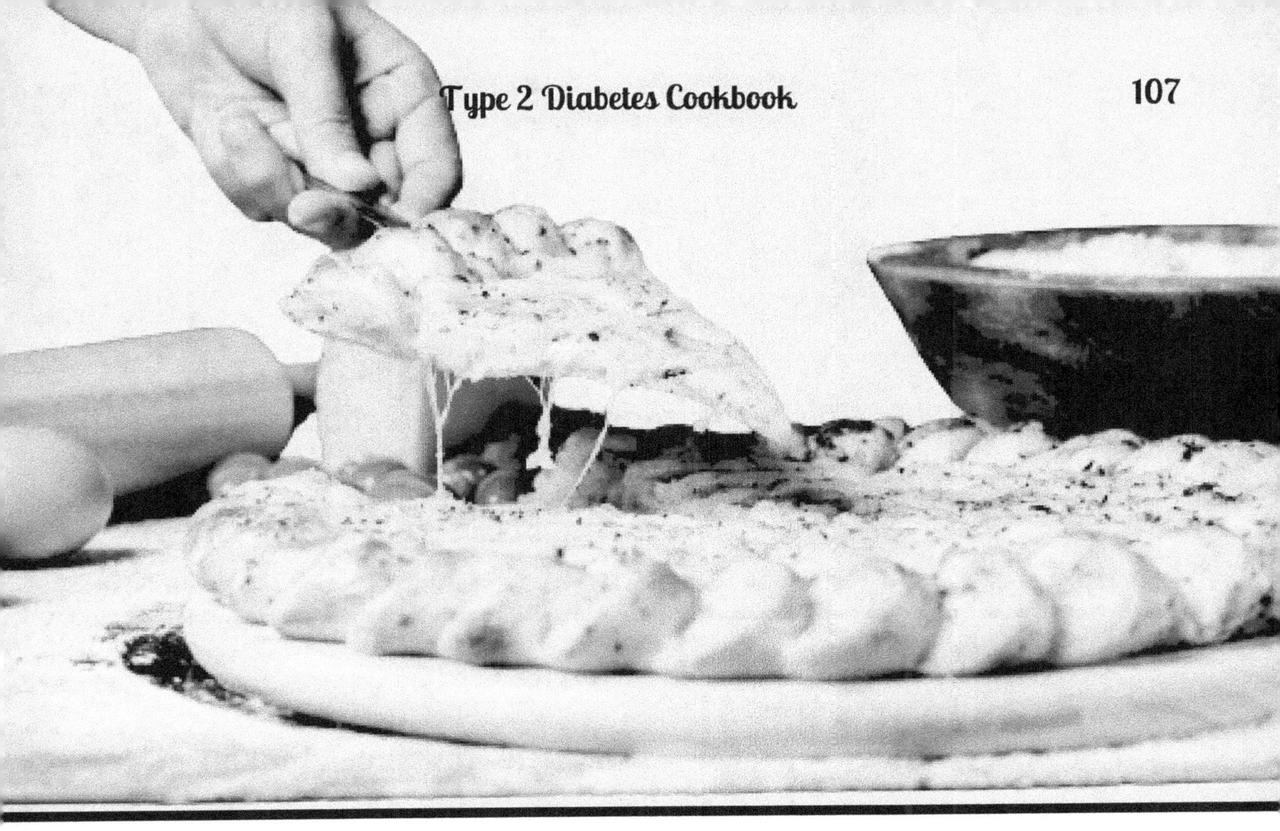

CHAPTER 12
DIABETIC COMFORT FOOD MAKEOVERS

Comfort foods can still be included in a diabetic-friendly diet. In this chapter, familiar favorites are revisited, giving them a healthy twist while retaining the warmth and satisfaction they offer. From the Healthier Chicken Alfredo with Zoodles to the Guilt-Free Apple Crisp, these recipes provide the comfort you crave while taking a mindful approach to diabetes management.

Healthier Chicken Alfredo: Zoodle perfection! 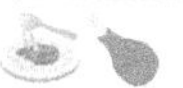

12.1 Healthier Chicken Alfredo with Zoodles

SERVES: 4   **PREP TIME: 15 MIN**   **COOKING TIME: 20 MIN**

INGREDIENTS

4 boneless, skinless chicken breasts

4 medium zucchinis, spiralized

2 tbsp olive oil

3 cloves garlic, minced

1 cup low-sodium chicken broth

1 cup unsweetened almond milk

1/2 cup grated Parmesan cheese

1 tbsp whole wheat flour

Salt and pepper to taste

Fresh parsley for garnish

DIRECTIONS

1. Season, grill, and slice chicken.
2. Sauté garlic in olive oil.
3. Sprinkle and whisk in flour.
4. Gradually add broth and almond milk, whisking until thick.
5. Stir in Parmesan until smooth.
6. Add zoodles, toss in Alfredo sauce.
7. Top with chicken strips.
8. Garnish with fresh parsley.

Note:
Healthier Chicken Alfredo with Zoodles transforms a classic indulgence into a diabetes-friendly delight. Zoodles replace traditional pasta, and the lighter Alfredo sauce keeps this comfort dish both satisfying and mindful.

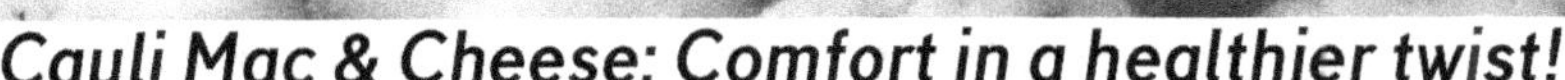

Cauli Mac & Cheese: Comfort in a healthier twist!

12.2 Cauliflower Mac & Cheese

SERVES: 6   PREP TIME: 201 MIN   BAKING TIME: 25 MIN

INGREDIENTS

1 medium cauliflower, cut into florets
8 oz whole wheat macaroni
1 cup unsweetened almond milk
1 1/2 cups sharp cheddar cheese, shredded
1/4 cup nutritional yeast
1 tsp Dijon mustard
1/2 tsp garlic powder
Salt and pepper to taste
Whole wheat breadcrumbs for topping
Chopped fresh parsley for garnish

DIRECTIONS

1. Preheat oven to 375°F (190°C); grease baking dish.
2. Cook cauliflower until tender; drain.
3. Cook macaroni; drain.
4. Blend almond milk, cheddar, nutritional yeast, mustard, garlic powder, salt, and pepper until smooth.
5. Mix macaroni, cauliflower, and cheese sauce in a bowl.
6. Transfer to baking dish, sprinkle breadcrumbs on top.
7. Bake 20-25 minutes until bubbly and golden.
8. Garnish with fresh parsley before serving.

Quick Sweet Potato Pie: Comfort food, pronto! 

12.3 Quick Sweet Potato Shepherd's Pie

SERVES: 6   **PREP TIME: 20 MIN**   **BAKING TIME: 25 MIN**

INGREDIENTS

2 lbs sweet potatoes, peeled and cubed
1/2 cup unsweetened almond milk
2 tbsp olive oil
1 onion, diced
2 carrots, diced
2 cloves garlic, minced
1 lb lean ground turkey
1 cup frozen peas
1 cup low-sodium chicken broth
1 tbsp tomato paste
1 tsp dried thyme
Salt and pepper to taste
Chopped fresh parsley for garnish

DIRECTIONS

1. Boil sweet potatoes until tender; mash with almond milk.
2. Sauté onion, carrots, and garlic in olive oil until softened.
3. Cook ground turkey until browned.
4. Stir in peas, chicken broth, tomato paste, thyme, salt, and pepper; simmer until peas are cooked.
5. Preheat oven to 375°F (190°C).
6. Transfer turkey mixture to a baking dish.
7. Spread mashed sweet potatoes on top.
8. Bake 20-25 minutes until golden.
9. Garnish with fresh parsley before serving.

Note: Sweet Potato Shepherd's Pie offers a comforting and diabetes-conscious twist on a classic dish.

Light Chicken Pot Pie: Comfort without the guilt! 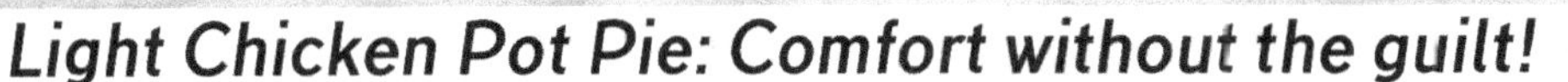

12.4 Lightened-Up Chicken Pot Pie

SERVES: 6   **PREP TIME: 20 MIN**   **BAKING TIME: 30-35 MIN**

INGREDIENTS

1 lb cooked, shredded chicken breasts
2 tbsp olive oil
1 onion, diced
2 carrots, diced
2 celery stalks, diced
2 cloves garlic, minced
1/4 cup whole wheat flour
2 cups unsweetened almond milk
1 cup low-sodium chicken broth
1 cup frozen peas
1 tsp dried thyme
Salt and pepper to taste
Whole wheat pie crust (store-bought or homemade)

DIRECTIONS

1. Preheat oven to 375°F (190°C); grease a pie dish.
2. Sauté onion, carrots, celery, and garlic in olive oil until softened.
3. Stir in whole wheat flour; cook for 2-3 minutes.
4. Gradually add almond milk and chicken broth; whisk until thickened.
5. Add shredded chicken, peas, thyme, salt, and pepper; stir.
6. Pour the mixture into the pie dish.
7. Roll out the whole wheat pie crust, place over filling, and seal edges.
8. Cut slits in the crust for steam.
9. Bake 30-35 minutes until golden.
10. Cool briefly before serving.

Lightened-Up Chicken Pot Pie gives a diabetic-friendly makeover to a classic comfort dish.

Guilt-Free Apple Crisp: Sweet indulgence, no regrets! 🍎

12.5 Guilt-Free Apple Crisp

SERVES: 6   **PREP TIME: 15 MIN**   **BAKING TIME: 40-45 MIN**

INGREDIENTS

6 cups Granny Smith apples, peeled and sliced

1 tablespoon lemon juice

1 teaspoon ground cinnamon

1/4 teaspoon nutmeg

1 cup rolled oats

1/2 cup almond flour

1/4 cup coconut oil, melted

1/4 cup maple syrup or sugar substitute

1/4 cup chopped walnuts

Vanilla Greek yogurt for serving

DIRECTIONS

1. Preheat oven to 350°F (175°C); grease a baking dish.
2. Toss sliced apples with lemon juice, cinnamon, and nutmeg.
3. Spread apples in the baking dish.
4. Combine oats, almond flour, melted coconut oil, maple syrup, and walnuts; sprinkle over apples.
5. Bake 40-45 minutes until golden and apples are tender.
6. Cool briefly before serving.
7. Serve with a dollop of vanilla Greek yogurt.

Note:

Guilt-Free Apple Crisp offers a diabetic-friendly alternative to a classic dessert. The combination of spiced apples and a wholesome oat topping creates a satisfying and guilt-free indulgence.

MEAL PLANNER

Sample

	BREAKFAST	LUNCH	DINNER	SNACK
DAY 1	Berry Bliss Bowl	Grilled Chicken Salad with Avocado Dressing	Baked Salmon with Lemon-Dill Sauce	Almond & Berry Energy Bites
DAY 2	Nutty Banana Bliss Oatmeal	Quinoa & Black Bean Power Bowl	Spaghetti Squash with Turkey Bolognese	Greek Yogurt & Berry Popsicles
DAY 3	Spinach & Feta Power Wrap	Zucchini Noodles with Pesto & Cherry Tomatoes	Chicken & Vegetable Stir-Fry	Veggie Sticks with Hummus
DAY 4	Classic Almond Flour Pancakes	Turkey & Vegetable Wrap	Herb-Crusted Tilapia	Nutty Trail Mix
DAY 5	Berry Blast Greek Yogurt Parfait	Cauliflower Fried Rice	Lentil & Vegetable Stew	Avocado & Tomato Salsa with Whole Grain Chips
DAY 6	Blueberry Bliss Almond Flour Pancakes	Salmon & Quinoa Stuffed Peppers	Roasted Vegetable Quinoa Bowl	Cucumber & Tuna Bites
DAY 7	Veggie-Packed Frittata Muffins	Spinach & Feta Turkey Burgers	Citrus-Marinated Grilled Chicken	Apples & Almond Butter Sandwiches

In
the pages that follow is a 28-day
Meal Planner. Feel free to customize
based on preferences and dietary
needs. Ensure a good balance of
macronutrients and portion sizes.
Adjust the plan to fit your lifestyle
and enjoy the variety of delicious,
diabetes-friendly meals!

Continue to mix and match recipes
from each chapter, ensuring a balance
of proteins, healthy fats, and complex
carbs. Integrate different cuisines and
flavors for variety. Consider
including dessert and snack options in
moderation.

28-DAY MEAL PLANNER

Week 1

	BREAKFAST	LUNCH	DINNER	SNACK
DAY 1				
DAY 2				
DAY 3				
DAY 4				
DAY 5				
DAY 6				
DAY 7				

WEEKLY MEAL PLANNER

Week 2

	BREAKFAST	LUNCH	DINNER	SNACK
DAY 8				
DAY 9				
DAY 10				
DAY 11				
DAY 12				
DAY 13				
DAY 14				

WEEKLY MEAL PLANNER

Week 3

	BREAKFAST	LUNCH	DINNER	SNACK
DAY 15				
DAY 16				
DAY 17				
DAY 18				
DAY 19				
DAY 20				
DAY 21				

WEEKLY MEAL PLANNER

Week 4

	BREAKFAST	LUNCH	DINNER	SNACK
DAY 22				
DAY 23				
DAY 24				
DAY 25				
DAY 26				
DAY 27				
DAY 28				

CONCLUSION

In finishing this voyage through the pages of "Type 2 Diabetic Cookbook and Meal Plan for the Newly Diagnosed," I sincerely hope that you have discovered not just a collection of recipes, but also a path to a more sustainable and happy diabetic existence. As we close up, let's go over the important diabetes-friendly cooking practices that have been incorporated into the fabric of this cookbook.

A recap of diabetes-friendly cooking techniques:

1. Mindful Carbohydrate Selection: Throughout this cookbook, I've stressed the significance of selecting complex carbohydrates over simple sweets. These options, ranging from whole grains to fiber-rich veggies, help to better manage blood sugar levels.

2. Portion Control: Every recipe was created with portion control in mind. By offering serving sizes, you can make informed choices about what goes on your plate.

3. Lean Protein Selections: Protein is an essential component of a diabetic-friendly diet. The cookbook provides a variety of lean protein sources, including turkey and chicken, fish, and plant-based options, to ensure a well-balanced and enjoyable meal.

4. Healthy Fats in Moderation: Incorporating healthy fats, such as those found in avocados, almonds, and olive oil, will help you eat a more balanced and tasty diet. The dishes strike a balance by encouraging the consumption of healthy fats in moderation.

5. Balanced Meal Planning: The meal plans supplied take a comprehensive approach to controlling type 2 diabetes. Each day is meticulously planned to give a balance of nutrients, flavors, and satisfaction while keeping blood sugar levels stable.

As you finish this cookbook, I hope you will believe that a diabetic-friendly lifestyle is not only manageable but also wonderfully fulfilling. Remember that you are not embarking on this path alone. You have the support of a community, the guidance of these recipes, and the inner fortitude to live a healthy and fulfilling life.

Here's to your health, happiness, and the beautiful trip that awaits.

Allison D. Dixon
Registered dietician and author